T0076569

Older Adults in Critical Care

Editor

DEBORAH GARBEE

CRITICAL CARE NURSING CLINICS OF NORTH AMERICA

www.ccnursing.theclinics.com

Consulting Editor
DEBORAH GARBEE

December 2023 • Volume 35 • Number 4

ELSEVIER

1600 John F. Kennedy Boulevard • Suite 1800 • Philadelphia, Pennsylvania, 19103-2899

http://www.theclinics.com

CRITICAL CARE NURSING CLINICS OF NORTH AMERICA Volume 35, Number 4
December 2023 ISSN 0899-5885, ISBN-13: 978-0-443-13101-1

Editor: Kerry Holland
Developmental Editor: Shivank Joshi

Critical Care Nursing Clinics of North America (ISSN 0899-5885) is published quarterly by Elsevier Inc., 360 Park Avenue South, New York, NY 10010-1710. Months of issue are March, June, September, and December. Business and Editorial Offices: 1600 John F. Kennedy Blvd., Suite 1800, Philadelphia, PA 19103-2899. Periodicals postage paid at New York, NY and additional mailing offices. Subscription prices are $160.00 per year for US individuals, $456.00 per year for US institutions, $100.00 per year for US students and residents, $206.00 per year for Canadian individuals, $573.00 per year for Canadian institutions, $230.00 per year for international individuals, $573.00 per year for international institutions, $115.00 per year for international students/residents and $100.00 per year for Canadian students/residents. To receive student/resident rate, orders must be accompanied by name of affiliated institution, data of term, and the *signature* of program/residency coordinator on institution letterhead. Orders will be billed at individual rate until proof of status is received. Foreign air speed delivery is included in all *Clinics* subscription prices. All prices are subject to change without notice. **POSTMASTER:** Send address changes to *Critical Care Nursing Clinics of North America*, Elsevier Health Sciences Division, Subscription Customer Service, 3251 Riverport Lane, Maryland Heights, MO 63043. **Customer Service: 1-800-654-2452 (US and Canada); 314-447-8871 (outside US and Canada). Fax: 314-447-8029. E-mail:** JournalsCustomerService-usa@elsevier.com **(for print support) and** JournalsOnlineSupport-usa@elsevier.com **(for online support).**

Reprints. For copies of 100 or more of articles in this publication, please contact the Commercial Reprints Department, Elsevier Inc., 360 Park Avenue South, New York, New York, 10010-1710; Tel.: 212-633-3874, Fax: 212-633-3820, and E-mail: reprints@elsevier.com.

Critical Care Nursing Clinics of North America is covered in *MEDLINE/PubMed (Index Medicus), International Nursing Index, Nursing Citation Index, Cumulative Index to Nursing and Allied Health Literature, and RNdex Top 100.*

Contributors

CONSULTING EDITOR

DEBORAH GARBEE, PhD, APRN, ACNS-BC, FCNS
Associate Dean Professional Practice, Community Service and Advanced Nursing
Practice, Program Director, Adult Gerontology Clinical Nurse Specialist Concentration,
Professor of Clinical Nursing, Louisiana State University Health Sciences Center School of
Nursing, The Louisiana Centre for Promotion of Optimal Health Outcomes: A JBI Centre of
Excellence, New Orleans, Louisiana

EDITOR

DEBORAH GARBEE, PhD, APRN, ACNS-BC, FCNS
Associate Dean Professional Practice, Community Service and Advanced Nursing
Practice, Program Director, Adult Gerontology Clinical Nurse Specialist Concentration,
Professor of Clinical Nursing, Louisiana State University Health Sciences Center School of
Nursing, The Louisiana Centre for Promotion of Optimal Health Outcomes: A JBI Centre of
Excellence, New Orleans, Louisiana

AUTHORS

MONCHIELLE BOLDS, MSN, RN, CNE
Instructor of Nursing, Louisiana State University Health Sciences Center New Orleans,
New Orleans, Louisiana

KATHRYN H. BOWLES, PhD, RN, FAAN, FACMI
University of Pennsylvania, University of Pennsylvania School of Nursing, Philadelphia,
Pennsylvania

CINNAMON BROOKE TUCKER, DNP, APRN, FNP, ACHPN
Louisiana and Mississippi Hospice and Palliative Care Association-Board Member, HPNA,
LANP, AANP, Palliative Medicine and Supportive Care, LCMC Health-University Medical
Center New Orleans, New Orleans, Louisiana

TERESA CRANSTON, MSN, RN, CCRN-K
Penn Medicine Lancaster General Hospital, Lancaster, Pennsylvania

JOSEPH EPPLING, DNP, MHA, RN, CRRN, NEA-BC
Louisiana State University Health Sciences Center New Orleans School of Nursing,
New Orleans, Louisiana

NOEL KOLLER-DITTO, DNP, APRN, AGCNS-BC
Assistant Professor, Eastern Michigan University, Ypsilanti, Michigan

QUINN LACEY, PhD, RN, CCRN
Louisiana State University Health Sciences Center New Orleans School of Nursing, New Orleans, Louisiana

REBEKAH LADUKE, MSN-NE, APRN, AG-ACCNS, CCRN
Critical Care Clinical Nurse Specialist, E.W. Sparrow Hospital, Lansing, Michigan

JENNIFER M. MANNING, DNS, ACNS-BC, CNE
Associate Dean for Undergraduate Nursing Programs, Louisiana State University Health Sciences Center New Orleans School of Nursing, New Orleans, Louisiana

MELISSA MARGUET, DNP, MBA, RN
Next Science LLC, Jacksonville, Florida

RACHEL NICKEL, BSN, MBA, RN, CCRN
University Medical Center New Orleans, New Orleans, Louisiana

COURTNEY NISSLEY, MS, RN, AGCNS-BC, CMSRN
Penn Medicine Lancaster General Hospital, Lancaster, Pennsylvania

MARY O'KEEFE, JD, PhD, APRN, CNS P/MH, LPC, FAAN
University of Texas Medical Branch at Galveston, Galveston, Texas

TRACY M. PARKER, MSN, APRN, FNP-BC
Nurse Practitioner in Acute and Outpatient Settings, Touro Heart and Vascular Care, LCMC Health, New Orleans, Louisiana

ELISSA PERSAUD, MSN, RN, ACCNS-AG, CCRN-CSC
Michigan Medicine, Ann Arbor, Michigan

ERIC PIASECKI, MSN, RN, APRN, ACCNS-AG, CCRN, TCRN, SCRN
Penn Medicine Lancaster General Hospital, Lancaster, Pennsylvania

DEBBRA POGUE, PhD, APRN, ACNS-BC, CCRN-K, CHSE
Our Lady of the Lake Regional Medical Center, Baton Rouge, Louisiana

CARRIE QUINN, MSN, RN, ACCNS-AG, CPAN, CNL-BC
Penn Medicine Lancaster General Hospital, Lancaster, Pennsylvania

MATTHEW REGULSKI, DPM, FFPM RCPS (Glasgow), ABMSP
Next Science LLC, Jacksonville, Florida; Medical Director, The Wound Care Institute of Ocean County, New Jersey

JENNIFER ROTTER, MSN, APRN, AGCNS-BC, CCRN-K
Quality Excellence Leader - Cardiovascular, Trinity Health Ann Arbor, Ypsilanti, Michigan

PATRICIA STEVENSON, DNP, APRN, CNS-C, CWS
Next Science LLC, Jacksonville, Florida

KATHARINE THOMPSON, BA, MSN, RN-BC, AGCNS-BC
Penn Medicine Lancaster General Hospital, Lancaster, Pennsylvania

CHLOÉ DAVIDSON VILLAVASO, MN, APRN, ACNS-BC, CV-BC, CMC, FPCNA, AACC
Clinical Faculty, Tulane University School of Medicine, Heart and Vascular Institute, New Orleans, Louisiana

SHAVONNE WILLIAMS, MN, APRN, ACNS-BC, ANVP-BC, SCRN, CCRN-K
Stroke Program Clinical Nurse Specialist, Texas Health Presbyterian Hospital, Dallas, Texas

NADINE WODWASKI, DNP, MSN-ed, ACNS, RN
Associate Professor, McAuley School of Nursing, University of Detroit Mercy, Detroit, Michigan

Contents

Having end-of-life (EOL) conversations is often difficult for even seasoned clinicians. There are many well-developed conversation guidelines used in the specialty of palliative medicine. There is no one ultimate guide that makes having an emotion-filled conversation easy. However, using the tenets of medical ethics, cloaked with experience, compassion, empathy, and respect makes EOL conversations less traumatic for the patient–family system and for the provider. Palliative specialists have the training and experience in effectively having EOL conversations, especially when death is unavoidable. Utilizing shared decision making, palliative specialists ensure there is mutual respect and communication between providers and the family system.

Engaging the health care team, including older adults and their caregivers, with the Institute for Healthcare Improvement 4M Model can help ensure every older adult receives (1) optimal health care, (2) is not harmed by health care, and (3) is satisfied with their health care. The evidence-based 4 Ms Model includes 4 significant concepts specific to older adult care: What matters, Mentation, Mobility, and Medication. Unfortunately, clinicians do not consistently apply the 4 M Model when caring for older adults. Personalized, age-friendly care based on the 4 M Model can improve outcomes for older adult patients.

Biofilm infections are a serious threat to public health, resistant to traditional treatments and host immune defenses. Biofilm infections are often polymicrobial, related to chronic wounds, medical devices (eg, knee replacements, catheters, tubes, contact lenses, or prosthetic valves) and chronic recurring diseases. Biofilms are more complex than nonadhered planktonic bacteria and produce a structure that prevents damage to the bacteria within the biofilm structure. The structure provides a hidden route to feed and nurture the bacteria allowing for ongoing spread of the bacteria.

Progressive supranuclear palsy (PSP) is a fatal neurodegenerative disorder. Care requires a patient-centered approach encompassing compassion, communication, and empathy. Despite concerted actions to streamline PSP patient transitions, the care is multifaceted and cause of concern. Patients with PSP undergoing transitional care are at an increased risk of undesirable outcomes, frequently endure poor communication, and encounter inconsistent care. Therefore, patients with PSP and families worry about the uncertainty in care, including who is accountable for the care and available resources. Through the three spheres of impact, Clinical Nurse Specialists can educate and assist intensive care unit nurses caring for patients with PSP /families, aiding in the successful care transition.

All patients within critical care units are vulnerable and many of them are unable to communicate their wishes and needs to the caregivers treating their acute critical illness. This inability to communicate is why interdisciplinary intensive care teams across the country heavily rely on spouses, children, siblings, parents, other next of kin, or other designated medical durable power of attorneys to advocate for those who cannot advocate for themselves. Unfortunately, there is a growing population of elder orphans who lack this support system when they need it the most.

A dedicated sepsis coordinator role at Penn Medicine Lancaster General Hospital led initiatives to improve sepsis core measure compliance by 40% during the course of 4 years with submission of all sepsis cases. Chart abstraction and analysis of noncompliant cases identified areas for improvement: early recognition education, order set revisions, documentation support, and the implementation of a nurse-driven 24/7 sepsis monitoring process. The cooperative work with Penn Medicine affiliates, sharing best practices, improves overall sepsis bundle compliance and transitions of care. Ongoing achievements acknowledge the value of building relationships and leading improvements through the collaborative efforts of interprofessional teams.

Elderly critical care patients are one of the largest growing patient population groups according to Medicare data. More than 51% of elderly patients are discharged on inappropriate medications that have the potential to cause harm or interact adversely with other medications. Precision health has the potential to prevent adverse drug events and prescription of inappropriate medications. The purpose of this literature review was to define the concept of precision health and determine the state of science regarding interprofessional models of precision health for assessment of caregiver impact on polypharmacy in elderly intensive care unit patients.

The demand for surgical intervention and hospitalization is expected to increase with the growth of the older adult population. Despite advances in technology and minimally invasive surgical procedures, the needs of the older adult in the perioperative period are unique. Transitions of care from the decision to support surgery through surgical intervention, subsequent hospitalization, and postacute discharge must be supported to achieve optimal patient outcomes. The clinical nurse specialist is well suited to address care delivery and assure implementation of best practices across the continuum.

Substance use disorders are increasing in the growing older adult population in the U.S. and abroad. Most interventions fail to account for the unique physical and psychosocial risk factors associated with substance use disorder. The older adult makes up a large portion of ICU admits and it is imperative to identify appropriate methods of prevention and treatment in this patient population. Important components of substance use disorder assessment and treatment in the older ICU patient were identified from the literature. Increased morbidity related to age-related conditions, pharmacologic concerns, withdrawals, and stigma were identified as essential items to consider when caring for the older ICU patient with substance use disorder.

Mental illnesses among critically ill patients are approximately 2.5 times that of the general population. Although older adults with physical–mental multimorbidity represent more than 50% of critical care admissions, health-care professionals caring for geriatric patients are not adequately educated to effectively recognize and treat serious mental illness. Additionally, critical care nurses feel vulnerable, unsupported, and unable to provide the best and safest possible patient-centered care for patients with mental illness. Hospitals can reduce these burdens by creating critical care policies and practices that are inclusive of geriatric and mental health concepts, care, and continuing education to those providing care.

Hospitals are always looking to improve the quality of patient care and avoid hospital-acquired conditions such as ventilator-associated pneumonia

(VAP). Currently, there are no set standards regarding interventions to prevent VAP, and there is not a single element that has a direct impact on VAP prevention. By creating an interprofessional team to work together, the quality improvement project was able to evaluate current practice compared with evidence-based practice in the literature to develop a critical care VAP bundle practice, which demonstrated improvement in compliance.

The cardiovascular geriatric population requiring intensive or critical care is a group vulnerable to adverse outcomes because of age, the critical care environment, geriatric syndromes, and multiple chronic conditions. Polypharmacy increases the risk of adverse events in this group. Several tools and aids are available to guide the clinical practice of appropriate prescribing and deprescribing. To optimize the care of the cardiovascular geriatric population, evidence-based prescribing, and deprescribing tools can be implemented by the interprofessional team consisting of the patient, their support system, critical care nurses, advanced practice clinicians, physicians, and allied health professionals.

Care models for older adults have been studied for more than 30 years. Several models of care for older adults were created in the acute care setting to prevent hospital-acquired disability and decline—a phenomenon frequently observed among older patients admitted in the acute care setting. The Acute Care for Elders (ACE) model and the Nurses Improving Care for Health System Elders program were 2 such models that sought to improve the quality of care for older adults and reduce their cost for care. Where are they today? Are we still using these care models in the acute care setting?

CRITICAL CARE NURSING
CLINICS OF NORTH AMERICA

SERIES OF RELATED INTEREST

Nursing Clinics of North America http://www.nursing.theclinics.com

THE CLINICS ARE AVAILABLE ONLINE!
Access your subscription at:
www.theclinics.com

Preface

Older Adults in Critical Care Settings

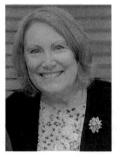

Deborah Garbee, PhD, APRN, ACNS-BC, FCNS
Editor

Older adults are admitted to critical care settings in increasing numbers that reflect growing numbers in the population. According to the US Census Bureau, one in six people in the United States are aged 65 or older, with the largest numbers in the 65- to 74-year age group.[1] In addition, the numbers in the 75- to 94-year age group grew slower, while the 95-year and older group had just below a 50% growth rate. Many older adults present with multimorbidity and frailty that compound health care needs. Multimorbidity, a diagnosis of greater than two morbidities, is frequently associated with poorer patient outcomes, higher health care costs, and decreased quality of life. It is estimated that more than 50% of older adults have three or more chronic conditions. With disease burden from multiple chronic conditions, older adults are prone to stress and psychological sequalae. Thus, the needs of older critical care patients range beyond the physical.

Frailty increases vulnerability of older adults in addition to their medical conditions. Frailty may be manifested by weakness, low physical activity, low energy, slow walking speed, and weight loss. Critical care nurses need to understand the connections between multimorbidity and frailty, as older adults comprise almost half of critical care admissions. Furthermore, the vulnerable older critical care patient may present with or without family support or a caregiver. The effects of education, low income, and environment impact overall health and well-being.

This issue of *Critical Care Nursing Clinics of North America* includes articles on (1) patient populations and care needs, such as incarcerated palliative care patients, progressive supranuclear palsy patients, and elder orphans; (2) models of care, for example, the 4M Model, ACE, and NICHE, and application of the precision health model; (3) bundled care outcomes, such as sepsis bundle, and ventilator-associated pneumonia; and (4)

Crit Care Nurs Clin N Am 35 (2023) xiii–xiv
https://doi.org/10.1016/j.cnc.2023.06.001
0899-5885/23/© 2023 Published by Elsevier Inc.

biofilm infections, transitions in care after general surgery, substance use disorders, geriatric psychiatry conditions of psychosis, delirium, depression, and suicide, and polypharmacy in cardiovascular patients.

Deborah Garbee, PhD, APRN, ACNS-BC, FCNS
Louisiana State University
Health Sciences Center
School of Nursing
1900 Gravier Street, 4A21
New Orleans, LA 70112, USA

E-mail address:
dgarbe@lsuhsc.edu

REFERENCE

1. United States Census Bureau (2023) 2020 Census: 1 in 6 people in the United States were 65 and over. Available at: https://www.census.gov/library/stories/2023/05/2020-census-united-states-older-population-grew.html. Accessed June 2, 2023.

Do We Really Listen, Improving End-of-Life Conversations

Cinnamon Brooke Tucker, DNP, APRN, FNP, ACHPN

KEYWORDS

- Palliative • End of life • Communication • Advanced practice registered nurse
- Incarcerated patients

KEY POINTS

- All clinicians should have primary palliative skills.
- Understanding when to consult a palliative care specialist.
- How to conduct an end-of-life conversation.
- Identifying a patient's goals of care.
- End of Life care while incarcerated.

INTRODUCTION

There are few things in life that we really get to "do over." Each person's death is an experience that is only lived once. Having practiced hospice and palliative care medicine for the past 20 years, this fact has never left the forefront of my medical decision-making and is a tenant of practice. Although people experience multiple deaths of family and friends throughout their lifetime, each one is a unique experience that is embedded into the memories of those left behind. As a provider, a patients' death may not be a life-altering moment, but for the patients and families we serve, death is personal and there are no second chances. Our profession also has trained us to code-switch and to move on unaffected to the next patient. This automation of practice leaves little time for grieving or debriefing by the health care professional.[1] Having the ability to sit with our own feelings about death and dying takes time, practice, resolve, and healing. To walk with a patient through a life-threatening illness or to embrace an inevitable death requires the provider to also have an acceptance of death and dying. Death, in this instance, is not a failure of the provider(s), giving up, or letting go of hope. Furthermore, death can be multifactorial, such as a loss of functional status, loss of good health, loss of role(s), and loss of relationship.[2]

Palliative Medicine and Supportive Care, LCMC Health-University Medical Center New Orleans, 2000 Canal Street, New Orleans, LA 70112, USA
E-mail address: Cinnamon.Tucker@LCMChealth.org

Crit Care Nurs Clin N Am 35 (2023) 357–365
https://doi.org/10.1016/j.cnc.2023.06.002
0899-5885/23/© 2023 Elsevier Inc. All rights reserved.

As clinicians in critical care, where life and death can be a moment away, we must be even more disciplined and efficient in having "difficult conversations." Why are the conversations difficult, I hypothesize that we have not been educationally and emotionally equipped to have these essential conversations. Just as we are taught to interpret laboratories and electrocardiograms (EKGs), we must also be trained to have effective end-of-life (EOL) conversations. Palliative care is not all about dying, but more so how to ensure patients live with complex chronic conditions or an acute life-threatening injury or illness.[3] All nurses, regardless of their specialty or level of education, should practice primary palliative medicine. This article aims to provide nurses with effective communication tools for EOL discussions including those with a vulnerable population, EOL incarcerated patients.

BACKGROUND

As a refresher, palliative to palliate means to "cloak" or cover to cover up: to "cover" the symptoms of illness without the intent to cure it. Care of the severely ill or dying can be found in ancient manuscripts and historical texts before the twentieth century. However, the concept of specialized care to the ill or dying was first documented in 1605 by Francis Bacon's proclamation that, "physicians should enable person to pass peacefully out of life," found in the book Palliative Care: The 400-year Quest for a Good Death.[4] More current, the modern hospice movement was started by British physician Dame Cicely Saunders in the 1960s. Inspired by Dr Saunders work, American nurse, Dr Florence Wald, became the mother of the American hospice movement. She spent time in London studying under Dr Saunders, eventually returned to Connecticut to open the first hospice program in 1974. Her work also expanded to prisons, creating a prison hospice program. In this program, inmates were trained to care for other inmates at the EOL.[5]

In 1975, the first palliative medicine program was established by Dr Balfour Mount. Later in 1987, Dr Declan Walsh established the first academic palliative program at the Cleveland Clinic. From there, palliative medicine rapidly expanded to hospitals across the country.[6] With a larger aging population, palliative care expanded its reach to patients who do not require hospitalization, yet still need specialized services of palliative medicine.[7]

Frameworks

Having the discussion is the most important fact, and having the conversations sooner rather than later, around the death bead, is most important. Palliative care as a specialty recommends conversations before illness or when a life-threatening illness is diagnosed. Unfortunately, the medical community still associates palliative care with hospice and death when it is really the opposite. Palliative care is about helping people LIVE with a serious illness until the very end. In some cases when appropriately consulted, some patients can return to their pre-illness state and no longer need the support of palliative care. How, when, and where you chose to discuss serious are secondary to just having the conversation.[3] What matters is that providers and patients are both talking and listening.

Three of the most widely used EOL frameworks that have been instrumental in developing effective EOL discussion are: "Ask, Tell, Ask," "What Matters Most," and "ABCDE." "Ask, Tell, Ask" guides a conversation creating a dialogue between patients and providers. The first "Ask" is to build trust; asking for permission to discuss, assessing for understanding, and asking about specific wishes regarding care such as medical proxy and code status. Next is the "Tell," the provider explains the condition in plain direct language that is compassionate and respectful. This phase of the conversation is when illness trajectory education and prognostic information is provided. We should not plan for our dying patients to fail by not preparing them for what to expect as the illness progresses. This may also be the appropriate time for a palliative care provider to educate the patient on transitioning back to primary providers, when a return to pre-illness state is likely. The patient should also be provided with information on how to manage their care moving forward. Specifically, for a palliative care provider, how you will manage symptoms and sojourner on the continuum of care. The final "Ask" is when the provider has the patient recall specifics regarding illness and prognosis.[8] For a video of how to perform an EOL conversation using "Ask, Tell, Ask", see Appendix A.

"What Matters Most" uses open-ended questions to initiate and elicit care goals: questions such as what kind of care would you want if you knew you were at the end of your life. The assumption should not be made that everyone wants to die at home surrounded by their families. *The Conversation Project* is an initiative of the Institute for Healthcare Improvement.[9] The communication is initiated by the provider and in some cases the health care proxy to allow the patient to openly discuss care goals that are based on their wishes. This guide is mostly used when the patient may be experiencing a sharp health decline, yet they are still verbal enough to express themselves clearly. This method can be used in an inpatient or outpatient setting. This approach can be very casual but also effective in understanding goals of care. For a video example of this approach, see (https://youtu.be/J1r0Xbh0UVo). There is also a free press document in multiple languages available to tailor to your institution or community. This document can be used as a living will, and embedded into the EHR, and shared across care teams. See Appendix B.

The "ABCDE" conversation framework is highly used worldwide and is used in emergent situations. This method has more closed-ended conversations that quickly and clearly identify the life-threatening illness or injury and assess goals of care. Answers are generally one word or one sentence responses. Often these conversations can be emotionally raw and heavy.

A—is for advanced preparation; it includes a full understanding of the clinical situation, checking your own emotional temperature, the setting in which the conversation will take place, and identifying the provider that should be involved in communication. The environment to have these conversations should be calm, private, and allow for family debriefing and further discussion.

B—is for build; building a therapeutic relationship and environment is paramount for effective discussion. Sit down, explain your role, learn who the person was before this event or what led to this event, ask for permission to speak openly, and what level of information should or should not be shared. Last, prepare the patient/family for what will happen next.[10]

C—means communication; use clear and concise information. After explaining bad news, allow space and time for silence. Keep a calm and professional tone should emotions and tension heighten. Ask follow-up questions to assess family understanding of the situation. Provide next steps such as who will speak with the patient, family next, when they will be able to see the patient, and when will the patient be seen again.[11]

D—stands for deal, dealing with the patient/family's emotions. Allow an environment for expression of emotions, watch body language. Answer any questions. Avoid mirroring the patient/family emotional response.[11] Actively listen to concerns, questions and validate the patient/family's emotions. Be genuine, compassionate, and empathetic. Enduring verbal abuse or disrespect from a patient or family is not ever acceptable.

E—is for emotions; encourage and validate the patient/family emotions. Provide supportive care. Answer any follow-up questions. Provide sympathy. No matter how poor the prognosis is, or if the extent of medical treatment has been exhausted, be honest, and offer another level of care, such as comfort focused care, home hospice, or inpatient hospice. Prepare the family if death is impending. Allow for open visitation and ongoing communication.[11]

In addition, there are two EOL communication packets that are immensely helpful, when immediate goals of care decisions are not essential, such as in the outpatient setting. *Five Wishes,* see Appendix C, and *The Conversation Project,* both give patients more independent time and control to decide on their goals of care. These guides can be extremely helpful in the outpatient setting.[9] The patient can take the packet home, and a follow-up appointment is made to discuss and embedded into the patient's plan of care. Special care must be provided to share the results of these documents with all members of the patient's treatment team. This can be challenging when a patient has multiple providers in various health systems or in private practice. Families should make copies of the Five Wishes and provide one to each of their providers. It is important for clinicians and families to understand that the Five Wishes is a living document; patients should be encouraged to ask their provider how the treatment plan aligns or intersects with the goals of care. The Five Wishes document can also be amended at any time.

As mentioned before, there are many conversation guidelines, and even scripts available. Scripts are useful for newer clinicians, an aid to help remain on task, and achieve objectives. They can also be a pitfall, when the situation is imminent, and emotions are high.

Listening to assess and understand the unique needs of each patient is vital to EOL conversations. Clinicians often come in with an agenda, leading the one-way communication, then asking if there are any questions at the end. In delivering "bad news," may patients do not hear anything beyond the bad news, they stop hearing, and their world starts spinning. When I am with my oncology patients, I always ask, "what did the oncologist say." Many times, the patient does not remember, and some are able to tell me the treatment plan. How often have we heard, "no one ever told me." I do believe the patient, and I believe my fellow providers. The provider was talking, and the patient was not listening. At the same time, the provider was talking and therefore not listening. "Patients have less anxiety, when they know their options".[12]

When to Consult Palliative Medicine

Palliative medicine is not a service of last resort. Modern palliative medicine should be engaged at any point and should be considered a partner in the delivery of health care services. Palliative medicine is available for all patients from the neonates in the neonatal intensive care unit (NICU) to the advanced centenarian. It is no longer just for those patients with cancer. Hospital-based and community-based palliative medicine services are expanding exponentially. However, the pervasive thought that palliative medicine is only for the dying, or those close to death, limits patients and families from the supportive care and symptom management so many patients' desperately need. Especially with a more aging population, these services should be a standard of care. Understandably, there is a lack of access to palliative care services. However, all clinicians should be prepared to manage general EOL conversations and basic symptom management.

To address the skeptics of why palliative medicine should not be consulted; (1) palliative does not take over care, on the contrary, palliative care does not provide primary care or seeks to discontinue the care provided by another specialist. (2) Palliative care as a specialty is not designed to be a feeder source for hospice enrollment. (3) Palliative care is not just emotional hand holding. Yes, palliative care providers, by design, are skilled communicators who use human care and touch to establish and maintain health care rapport with patients. (4) Palliative care is only needed when patients and families are labeled difficult. Often, patients and families are labeled difficult because of medical mistrust, lack of mutual respect and understanding, and having unmet medical and psychiatric needs. (5) Provider burnout is real, and managing patient care in silos does not ultimately meet the needs of the patient and is not sustainable long term. (6) Palliative medicine is not chronic pain management. Last, palliative care does encompass hospice, but hospice does not encompass palliative.[13]

Palliative Medicine for Incarcerated Patients

The institution where I am employed has a state contract to provide care to incarcerated persons, for inpatient and outpatient services. The Department of Corrections (DOC) has access to our EHR, and their case managers and medical units have full access to patient information for care coordination. This was my first experience as a palliative care provider that I worked closely with incarcerated persons. Before this experience, I was sorely unaware of the unique needs, challenges, and complexities of care of the incarcerated. From my previous experience as a hospice provider and watching documentaries on prison hospices, I knew that hospice care was available at some prisons. However, I did not know the amount of care coordination and social-emotional implications of palliative care at EOL for incarcerated patients.

The first compassionate release case I managed was a 42-year-old man with pancreatic cancer. Unfortunately, he suffered multiple complications leading to an extended hospitalization and was no longer walking or eating. My medical director suggested that I start the process of filing for a compassionate release. Within 2 weeks, the paperwork, video, and statement of prognosis were sent to the DOC, and he was released. He was moved from the closed access unit (also known as the prison unit) to a regular patient room. His family was then allowed to visit and his condition slightly improved. The hospice agency brought equipment and medications to his family's home in anticipation of hospital discharge. I thought it was a win for the patient until he was remanded back into custody and taken to a maximum security prison medical unit. Everyone involved, including myself, was shocked. Unbeknownst to me, multiple layers of detail are needed for a compassionate release, and there are no guarantees.

Just as our society ages and has higher utilization of health care; the prison population also ages and has higher health care costs due to health disparities associated with incarcerated persons. Ninety percent of deaths in prisons are patients more than the age of 65 years that have multiple chronic conditions.[14] The health care age of a person incarcerated is 10 years older than their chronologic age. Incarcerated individuals have higher rates of lung and hepatic cancers and have shorter survival rates compared with the general population.[15] Many misconceptions exist in care of the incarcerated. To start, persons incarcerated have a constitutional right to standard health care. One would think that extends to palliative and EOL care. However, the most recent data demonstrate that there are almost 7000 jails in the United States, incarcerating almost 2 million people.[16] Yet, there are only 75 prison hospice facilities in the United States. There were no documented findings of palliative care specialists in the prison system.[14]

One of the many ways health care providers are addressing the EOL needs in the incarcerated populations is when the person presents for health care external to the prison system. Hospitals that contract with local prisons and jails should seek to address advanced care planning on entry into the health care system. A study done within a prison contracted hospital, palliative medicine was only consulted in 45% (*n* = 136) of the patients who died, furthermore individuals did not receive a palliative care consult until 3 days before death. Of 45%, goals of these cases were the trigger for consult in only 50% of those cases.[14] Furthermore, clinicians must also be educated on health care rights of those incarcerated. Relying on oral traditions and misconceptions are further adding to the disparities of an already vulnerable population.

With almost half of incarcerated patients receiving palliative care consults in the last week of life begs the question of who is providing and meeting patient care and support needs. **Fig. 1** offers insight into a possible answer to this question, yet introduces more questions related to support for the caregiver.

Any patient diagnosed with a serious illness or life-threatening injury, which is appropriate for palliative care, should be evaluated for a compassionate release. Palliative care consultant services are your partners in the care of incarcerated patients outside of the prison health care system. Consultant services in many cases have formalized relationships established with prisons. Palliative care providers are aware of processes to ensure there is effective communication between the hospital, prison, DOC, and the families. Many times, if a process is initiated while the patient is in the hospital, the release often does not happen during the acute stay. Patients may return to their prison of record or a different prison medical unit depending on their care needs. Palliative care providers can also follow patients that are not yet medically eligible for release due to high functional status and active treatment. Palliative care teams remain consistent within an institution, whereas treatment teams may vary. Palliative care provides an essential link in care coordination to have ongoing communication with prison medical providers, oncologists, intensivists, and other specialists.

In institutions without the benefit of palliative care consultant services, documentation of conversations with prison officials, petitions for release documentation, and care team communication are imperative. This documentation should not be

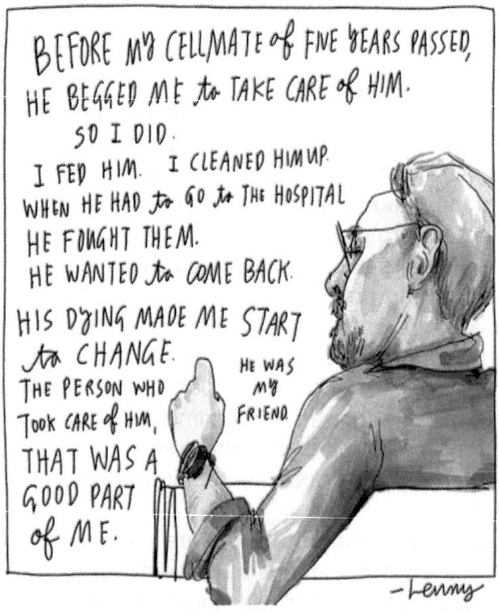

Fig. 1. Incarcerated palliative care patient support.

embedded solely within treatment notes. Stand-alone documentation notes should be created within the EHR. Communication flags within the health record are also another method of identification. Any step to advocate for the compassionate release of an individual is important.

SUMMARY

EOL conversations should not be difficult; it just takes practice and time. Using any of the frame works discussed or creating your own blend is helpful, the important thing to remember is to be genuine, compassionate, and empathetic. Listen to understand, and just as we have patients recall what was taught, as the clinician, ensure you are hearing what is most important to the patient and family. Be prepared, set the environment, and speak in a language that is relatable to your patient. Consider advancing your knowledge and obtain certification in hospice and palliative medicine (www.hpna.org). If you do not have a palliative care consultant service, you can become a palliative care champion within your organization, regardless of your specialty. When incarcerated individuals are in your care, remember to discuss advanced care planning. It is never too early to consult palliative medicine or initiate advanced care planning discussions. Palliative consultants can be found in hospital and clinic-based settings, telehealth services, and have now expanded to community-based settings, offering home-based care. In the words of Mother Theresa, "No one person can do everything, but everyone can do something."

CLINICS CARE POINTS

- It is never too early to discuss advance care planning.
- All clinicians should have basic primary palliative care skills.
- Use end-of-care (EOL) frameworks to guide your discussions.
- Palliative care is not hospice; avoid using the terms interchangeably.
- Early consultation improves patient outcomes and increases patient–provider satisfaction.
- Goals of care documents are living documents that are modifiable at any time.
- Listening to assess and understand the unique needs of each patient is vital to EOL conversations.
- Palliative medicine is for all patients from the neonate to the centenarian.
- Some patients are "too sick to live" and death is not a necessary failure.
- Debrief frequently and allow for self-care.
- Clinicians need education on unique needs, challenges, and complexities of care of the incarcerated palliative care patient.

DISCLOSURE

There are no commercial or financial conflicts of interest.

REFERENCES

1. Larson D, Tobin D. End-of-life conversations: evolving practice and theory. JAMA 2000;284(12):1573–8.

2. Mistry B, Bainbridge D, Bryant D, et al. What matters most for end-of-life care? from community-based palliative care providers and administrators. BMJ Open 2015;5:e007492.

3. Radwaney, S. Finding calm in the storm: A palliative care approach to navigating the family meeting. NHPCO-Palliative Care Series.https://www.nhpco.org/wpcontent/uploads/2019/04/PALLIATIVECARE_CalmInStorm.pdf. Date Assessed: April 7, 2023.

4. Piana R. A History of medical care for the dying.https://ascopost.com/issues/may-10-2016/a-history-of-medical-care-for-the-dying/.Date Accessed: March 24, 2023.

5. American Association for the History of Nursing. (2018) https://www.aahn.org/wald_f. Date Accessed: February 18, 2023.

6. Tatum P, Craig W, Washington K, et al. Getting comfortable with death. Evolution of the care of the dying patient. Mo Med 2014;111(4):298–303.

7. Hughes M, Smith T. The growth of palliative care in the United States. Annu Rev Publ Health 2014;35(1):459–75.

8. Bernacki R, Block S. Communication about serious illness care goals: a review and synthesis of best practices. JAMA Intern Med 2014;174(12):1994–2003.

9. Institute for Healthcare Improvement. The conversation project. Available at:https://theconversationproject.org/videos. Accessed 1 April, 2023.

10. Astier A. How to use the ABCDE framework for delivering bad or life-altering news, 2021, Educating in Medicine & Pharmacy, Available at: https://www.andreasastier.com/blog/how-to-use-the-abcde-framework-for-delivering-bad-or-life-altering-news. Accessed April 4, 2023.

11. Bagley J. Delivering difficult patient conversations is a skill to be learned and practiced, *American College of Surgeons*, 108 (2), 2023, Available at: https://www.facs.org/for-medical-professionals/news-publications/news-and-articles/bulletin/2023/february-2023-volume-108-issue-2/delivering-difficult-patient-conversations-is-a-skill-to-be-learned-practiced/. Accessed April 4, 2023.

12. Anglin A. Break bad news to patients with this step-by-step guide. ONS Voice; 2022. https://voice.ons.org/news-and-views/break-bad-news-to-patients-with-this-step-by-step-guide. Accessed: April 7, 2023.

13. Buss M, Rock I, McCarthy E. Understanding palliative care and hospice: a review for primary care providers. Mayo Clin Proc 2017;92(2):280–6. https://www.sciencedirect.com/science/article/abs/pii/S0025619616307637. Assessed: March 23, 2023.

14. DiThomas, M. & Williams, B. (2022). Palliative care for incarcerated adults. UpToDate.https://www.uptodate.com/contents/palliative-care-for-incarcerated-adults. Date Accessed: March 1, 2023.

15. Stephens S, Cassel B, Noreika D, et al. Palliative care for inmates in the hospital setting, *Am J Hospice Palliat Med*, 36 (4), 2019, 321–325, Available at: pubmed.ncbi.nlm.nih.gov/30428682/. Accessed March 1, 2023.

16. Sawyer W, Wagner P. Mass incarcerations: The whole pie 2023. Prison Policy Initiative. https://www.prisonpolicy.org/reports/pie2023.html#:~:text=Together%2C%20these%20systems%20hold%20almost,centers%2C%20state%20psychiatric%20hospitals%2C%20and. Date Accessed: March 30, 2022.

APPENDIX

Appendix A. UCFS. ePrognosis.

Communication Skills: Ask Tell Ask. ePrognosis - Communication (ucsf.edu) Date retrieved: May 31, 2023.

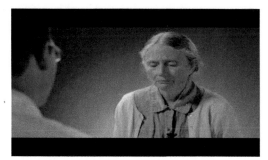

Appendix B. The Conversation Project Handout.

The Conversation Project - Have You Had The Conversation? Accessed April 1, 2023.

Appendix C. Five Wishes.

https://www.fivewishes.org/five-wishes-sample.pdf Date Accessed April 1, 2023.

The 4M Model

Jennifer M. Manning, DNS, ACNS-BC, CNE

KEYWORDS

- 4M model • Age-friendly health systems • Health care • Older adults

KEY POINTS

- Engaging the health care team, including older adults and their caregivers, with the 4M Model can help ensure every older adult receives optimal health care, is not harmed by health care, and is satisfied with their health care.
- The evidence-based 4 M Model includes 4 major concepts specific to older adult care: What Matters, Mentation, Mobility, and Medication.
- Clinicians are not consistently applying the 4 M Model when determining care for older adults.
- Personalized, age-friendly care based on the 4 M Model can improve clinical outcomes for older adult patients.

INTRODUCTION

Older adults are an increasingly important demographic, as people worldwide live longer than ever, increasing from 66.8 years in 2000 to 73.4 years in 2019.[1] The number of older adults is expected to double by 2050.[1] In addition, older adults experience more chronic conditions, complex health care needs, and severe illnesses than younger adults. With this increase in life expectancy, the health and well-being of older adults have become a key point of emphasis for health care providers and policy-makers. An estimated 41.8 million Americans were caregivers of an older adult in 2020; this number is estimated to increase with the increasing older adult population.[1]

Approximately 77% of older adult Americans have 2 or more chronic conditions. Older adults are eligible for benefits such as Medicare and Medicaid health care coverage.[2] Older adult Medicare recipients visit at least 2 primary care providers and 5 specialists annually to manage chronic conditions. Unfortunately, many health care providers do not communicate together, leading to the fragmentation of care for older adults. Subsequently, older adults experience more emergency room visits and hospitalizations.[2] The care hospital-based teams provide does not reflect older adults' unique needs. When admitted to the hospital, older adults, especially those with cognitive impairment, are at increased risk for declining mobility, falls, malnutrition, and

Louisiana State University Health Sciences Center School of Nursing, 1900 Gravier Street, New Orleans, LA 70112, USA
E-mail address: Jmanni@lsuhsc.edu

Crit Care Nurs Clin N Am 35 (2023) 367–374
https://doi.org/10.1016/j.cnc.2023.06.003
0899-5885/23/© 2023 Elsevier Inc. All rights reserved.
ccnursing.theclinics.com

delirium, extending the length of stay and leading to poor health outcomes.[2] Caregivers and providers must apply evidence-based research to promote high-quality care for older adults. To best support the needs of older adults, it is essential to have a model for understanding the unique challenges and opportunities they face. One such model is the 4M model, designed to address the specific needs of older adults.[3]

The Institute for Healthcare Improvement 4M model

The John A. Hartford Foundation and the Institute for Healthcare Improvement (IHI) partnered with the American Hospital Association and Catholic Health Association of the United States to develop an Age-Friendly Health System initiative aimed at ensuring older adults receive optimal health care—the initiative called for implementing the 4 Ms of an Age-Friendly Health System, an evidence-based model.[2,3]

The 4M model is based on a foundation of existing geriatric care models and provides a structure for the health care team to organize care (**Fig. 1**). Each aspect of the model is incorporated into daily health care practice. The key is to assess and act on these aspects for each older adult at the point of care and recognize that each of the 4 Ms impacts the other areas.[3]

Caregivers implementing the 4M model are critical to ensure optimal care. The 4M model is an approach to care that focuses on 4 key areas: What Matters, Medication, Mentation, and Mobility.[4] Each of these areas is critical to the health and well-being of older adults, and together they provide a comprehensive approach to caring for this population. The model is intended to be used with every older adult during every health care interaction across settings and transitions in care. Currently, more than 600 hospitals and health care practices are recognized by IHI as Age-Friendly Health Systems implementing the 4M model.[5] Each of the 4M concepts is described in more detail and discusses how the 4M model can support older adults' health and well-being.

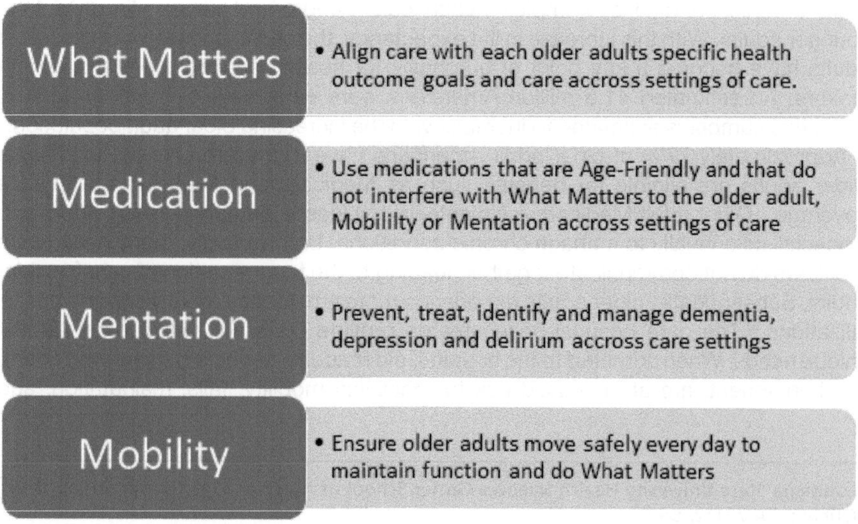

What Matters	• Align care with each older adults specific health outcome goals and care accross settings of care.
Medication	• Use medications that are Age-Friendly and that do not interfere with What Matters to the older adult, Mobililty or Mentation accross settings of care
Mentation	• Prevent, treat, identify and manage dementia, depression and delirium accross care settings
Mobility	• Ensure older adults move safely every day to maintain function and do What Matters

Fig. 1. The institute for health care improvement 4M model. (Reference: Institute for Healthcare Improvement (IHI). Age-friendly health systems guide to using the 4 Ms in the care of older adults. https://www.ihi.org/Engage/Initiatives/Age-Friendly-Health-Systems/Documents/IHI AgeFriendlyHealthSystems_GuidetoUsing4MsCare.pdf.)

What Matters

The "What Matters" concept is an important starting point for implementing the 4M Model.[5] "What Matters" includes assessing what is essential to the older adult's health care and personal lives (**Fig. 2**). Then, the health care team can align the care plan to the older adults' goals and preferences. Areas of importance commonly included in "What Matters" to the older adult include managing pain preferences, maintaining social connections with family and friends, and returning to baseline activities. In addition, in the hospital setting, it is vital to ask the older adult what they hope for during this hospitalization.[6]

Once it is known "What Matters," the clinician can ensure the health care team knows "What Matters" and align the care plan accordingly. Furthermore, caregivers can be crucial in communicating preferences during shift reports and rounds to keep the health care team informed. Finally, caregivers are essential in advocating for the older adult and ensuring choices are addressed.[6]

Medications

Medications are a critical component of health care for many older adults, as they can help to manage chronic conditions and improve overall health. However, medications can also pose significant risks to older adults, mainly when multiple medications are used or not as prescribed. Therefore, the 4M model emphasizes the importance of medication management to improve the health and well-being of older adults.[5]

Several strategies can be used to improve medication management in older adults. One critical approach is to review the medications a patient takes regularly to identify any potential interactions or side effects. A health care provider or pharmacist can do this, which may involve changing the patient's medication regimen.[6]

Another critical strategy for medication management is to ensure that medications are being taken as prescribed. Medication management may involve medication reminders or other tools to help patients remember to take their medications. Additionally, health care providers may need to adjust medication dosages or change medications if side effects or interactions are identified.[5]

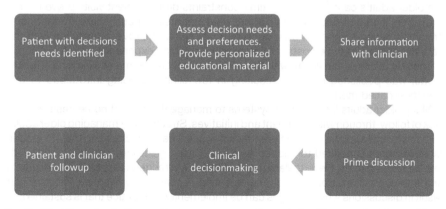

Fig. 2. Workflow for better patient engagement through health care decision-making. (Reference: IHI. Age-friendly health systems guide to using the 4 Ms in the care of older adults. https://www.ihi.org/Engage/Initiatives/Age-Friendly-Health-Systems/Documents/IHI AgeFriendlyHealthSystems_GuidetoUsing4MsCare.pdf.)

Mentation

Mentation refers to cognitive function, including memory, attention, and decision-making. Cognitive decline is a common concern for older adults and can significantly impact their quality of life. Therefore, the 4M model emphasizes the importance of addressing mentation issues to improve older adults' health and well-being.[5]

Many strategies can be used to improve mentation in older adults. One integral approach is cognitive training, which involves engaging in activities challenging cognitive function. Cognitive training improves cognitive function in older adults, particularly in areas such as memory and attention. Other strategies for improving mentation in older adults include addressing underlying conditions such as depression or anxiety.[6]

Mobility

Mobility is a crucial concern for older adults, as physical limitations can significantly impact their quality of life. Mobility issues can arise from various factors, including chronic conditions such as arthritis, injuries such as falls, and changes in vision or hearing. The 4M model emphasizes the importance of addressing mobility issues to improve the health and well-being of older adults.[5]

Many strategies can be used by clinicians to improve mobility in older adults.[5] One integral approach is exercise, which has been shown to improve strength, balance, and flexibility in older adults. In particular, resistance training has been offered to improve mobility in older adults with mobility limitations effectively.[6] Other strategies for improving mobility include assistive devices such as canes or walkers, modifications to the home environment, and physical therapy.[5]

In addition to the mobility interventions described, addressing the underlying causes of mobility issues in older adults is essential. For example, managing chronic conditions such as arthritis or osteoporosis can help to improve mobility in these patients. Similarly, addressing vision and hearing issues can help to improve balance and reduce the risk of falls.[6,7]

Barriers to Adopt the 4M Model

There are barriers to adopting the 4M model. These barriers center around inadequate planning and integration into practice. For example, most clinicians do not routinely ask older adults "What Matters," nor do they align care plans with what matters in the older adult's care.[7] Clinicians' time constraints during patient visits prevent clinicians from incorporating questions about what matters into patient care. Furthermore, engaging patients in health care decision-making can improve satisfaction with the care experience, reduce costs, and benefit the clinician experience.[8,9]

There is a lack of familiarity with the 4M approach among many clinicians. The 4M model was published recently, resulting in few clinicians being introduced to this evidence-based model.

Many older adults lack support systems to manage the 4 Ms at home, resulting in a lack of follow-through with treatment and initiatives. Strategies for managing older adults with few social support systems create challenges when implementing the 4M model. More research is needed to support evidence-based guidelines for older adults with few support systems. Nevertheless, integrating the 4M model is feasible for older adults and improves clinical outcomes. Implementing a quality improvement initiative can result in discussions when changes can be implemented in practice that is sustained.[6,8]

Resources for Clinicians and Caregivers

There are multiple resources and tools available to assess and address the 4 Ms (**Table 1**). For example, to determine what matters, tools such as VitalTalk can support

Table 1
A resource to implement the 4M model

4 Ms	Look for How the Organization Does the Following	Current Organization Practice
What Matters: Aligning care with every older adult's specific health outcome goals and care preferences across settings of care	• Align older adult care plan with What Matters Most • Ask the older adult What Matters, then document and share with the health care team	\<add information here\>
Medication: If medication is necessary, use age-friendly medication that does not interfere with What matters to the older adult, their mobility or mentation across care settings	• Review high-risk medications and document • Adjust high-risk medications and avoid use when possible	\<add information here\>
Mentation: Prevent, treat, and manage dementia, depression, and delirium across care settings	Hospital • Screen for delirium every 12 h and document • Provide oral hydration • Orient to time, place, and situation • Ensure older adults have adaptive equipment • Prevent interruptions in sleep, use nonpharmacological interventions to support sleep Ambulatory • Screen for cognitive impairment and document results • If experiencing cognitive impairment, refer for evaluation and manage in the health care setting • Screen for depression and document • If experiencing depression, identify and manage contributing factors. Refer for treatment	\<add information here\>
Mobility: Ensure each older adult moves safely to maintain function and do what matters	• Screen for mobility limitations and document • Ensure early, frequent, and safe mobility	\<add information here\>

(Reference: IHI. Age-friendly health systems guide to using the 4 Ms in care of older adults. https://www.ihi.org/Engage/Initiatives/Age-Friendly-Health-Systems/Documents/IHIAgeFriendlyHealthSystems_GuidetoUsing4MsCare.pdf.)

communication. In addition, VitalTalk includes evidence-based training for clinicians, faculty, and organizations to equip clinicians, educators, and organizations in providing patient-centered care.[10] Clinician development in communication is a critical skill necessary to provide high-quality patient care.

For the medications portion of the 4M model, a helpful resource for deprescribing is www.deprescribing.org. Deprescribing is part of good prescribing for older adult patients. When clinicians back off of older adult medication high doses or stop medications that are no longer needed, there is a reduction in the risk of drug-related harm to the patient. This website offers information for providers, such as evidence-based deprescribing guidelines, the process used for developing deprescribing guidelines, and the steps to carry safe prescribing for an older adult patient.[10,11]

The American Geriatrics Society (AGS) CoCare Hospital Elder Life Program (HELP) is an evidence-based model of hospital care designed to prevent functional decline and delirium. This model is a helpful resource for addressing the mentation concept in the 4M model. The program integrates principles of geriatrics into standard nursing and medical care while bringing older adult expertise into the patient care decisions.[10] The HELP program has been shown to reduce the onset and prevention of delirium, prevent functional decline, improve the overall quality of hospital care for older adult patients, and reduce hospital costs for older adults.[12,13]

The Centers for Disease Control and Prevention (CDC) Preventing Falls Guide is a helpful resource for improving mobility. This "how to" guide is designed for organizations implementing evidence-based fall prevention programs. The Falls Guide provides guidelines on program planning, development, implementation, and evaluation.[12] In addition, the guide addresses questions important when implementing fall prevention programs, such as finding a program that meets the needs of older adult patients, what resources and support are needed, what partners should help with program development, and how to sustain the program for future use.[14,15]

Recommendations for Applying the 4M Model in Critical Care Settings

Older adults represent the vast expanding population in critical care units. Caring for older adults in critical care settings is challenging due to multiple factors such as comorbidities, polypharmacy, frailty, and advance directives. Once admitted, tailoring safe treatment plans to match the older adults' wishes and personalized needs will guide critical care for the older adult patient. The 4M model can be applied in critical care settings during assessment and care transitions.

During an assessment, the 4M model can be applied in critical care settings to identify patients who would benefit from a geriatric clinician referral. Referral can be based on assessment findings from the 4M concepts of what matters, mentation, mobility, and medication. For example, a positive Confusion Assessment Method (CAM) Score, recent fall history, positive medication screen based on the Beers list, lack of an advanced directive, or an undocumented code status all indicate the need for further referral.[16,17]

During transitions of care, the 4M model can be used to identify patients at risk for further illness or injury. For example, suppose the need for a referral for physical therapy, occupational therapy or social work is recognized. In that case, a referral can be initiated acutely and continue during the care transitions through follow-up with the clinician post-discharge. It is critical to note that automating the referral process is key to ensuring older adult patients are not lost during the follow-up or re-hospitalization phase and to ensure a full understanding of discharge instructions.[16,17]

SUMMARY

The American population is experiencing a shift to more older adults. In 2034, the older adult population will outnumber children for the first time in US history. In addition, the United States is also becoming more racially and ethnically diverse, with non-Hispanic white people becoming the minority population. Health care delivery will have to evolve to meet the demographic population shifts. Health care clinicians must be skilled in assessing older adults' needs, values, and preferences to create a foundation for an age-friendly approach to managing their chronic conditions, care coordination, and medication adherence. Presently, the education of health care clinicians lacks a uniform focus on reliable content related to the 4M model. This approach can support health care clinicians in developing consistent assessment strategies and using resources to improve older adult patient care.

CLINICS CARE POINTS

- Once admitted to a critical care setting, tailoring safe treatment plans to match the older adults' wishes and personalized needs will guide critical care interventions for the older adult patient.
- The 4M model can be applied to older adult patients in critical care settings during assessment and care transitions.
- During an assessment of the older adult patient, the 4M model can be applied in critical care settings to identify who would benefit from a geriatric clinician referral.
- Referral can be based on assessment findings from the 4M concepts of what matters, mentation, mobility, and medication.
- During transitions of care, the 4M model can identify patients at risk for further illness or injury.

REFERENCES

1. Ortman JM, Velkoff VA, Hogan H, et al. An aging nation: the older population in the United States: population estimates and projections, 2014, US Census Bureau; Washington, DC, P25-1140. Current population reports: Available at: https://www.census.gov/library/publications/2014/demo/p25-1140.html#:~:text=In%202050%2C%20the%20population%20aged,over%20the%20age%20of%2085.
2. Cacchione PZ. Age-friendly health systems: the 4Ms framework. Clin Nurs Res 2020;29(3):139–40.
3. Lesser S, Zakharkin S, Louie C, et al. Clinician knowledge and behaviors related to the 4Ms framework of age-friendly health systems. J Am Geriatr Soc 2022; 70(3):789–800.
4. Emery-Tiburcio EE, Mack L, Zonsius MC, et al. The 4Ms of an Age-Friendly Health System an evidence-based framework to ensure older adults receive the highest quality care. Home Healthc Now 2022;40(5):252–7.
5. IHI. Age friendly health systems guide to using the 4Ms in care of older adults. Available at: https://www.ihi.org/Engage/Initiatives/Age-Friendly-Health-Systems/Documents/IHIAgeFriendlyHealthSystems_GuidetoUsing4MsCare.pdf.
6. Avallone M, Perweiler E, Pacetti S. Using the 4Ms framework to teach geriatric competencies in a community clinical experience. Nurs Forum 2021;56(1):83–8.

7. Dolansky MA, Pohnert A, Ball S, et al. Pre-implementation of the age-friendly health systems evidence-based 4ms framework in a multi-state convenient care practice. Worldviews Evid Based Nurs 2021;18(2):118–28.

8. Krist AH, Tong ST, Aycock RA, et al. Engaging patients in decision-making and behavior change to promote prevention. Stud Health Technol Inform 2017;240: 284–302.

9. Guth A, Chou J, Courtin SO, et al. An interdisciplinary approach to implementing the age-friendly health system 4ms in an ambulatory clinical pathway with a focus on medication safety. J Gerontol Nurs 2020;46(10):7–11.

10. Learn to Communicate Effectively with Patients Living with Serious Illnesses. Vital Talk. Accessed June 1, 2023. About Us - VitalTalk.

11. Mack L, Zonsius MC, Newman M, et al. Recognizing and acting on mentation concerns. Am J Nurs 2022;122(5):50–5.

12. AGS CoCare: Hosptial Elder Life Program (HELP). American Geriatrics Society CoCare. Accessed June 1, 2023. AGS CoCare - Help.

13. Olson LM, Zonsius MC, Rodriguez-Morales G, et al. Promoting safe mobility. Am J Nurs 2022;122(7):46–52.

14. Olson LM, Zonsius MC, Rodriguez-Morales G, et al. Promoting Safe Mobility Strategies for partnering with caregivers to maximize older adults' functional ability. Home Healthc Now 2023;41(2):105–11.

15. Older Adult Fall Prevention. Centers for Disease Control and Prevention. 2023. Older Adult Falls | Fall Prevention | Injury Center | CDC.

16. Megalla M, Avula R, Manners C, Chinnery P, et al. Using the 4M model to screen geriatric patients in the emergency department. Journal of Geriatric Emergency Medicine 2021;2(9). Available at: https://gedcollaborative.com/jgem/using-the-4m-model-to-screen-geriatric-patients-in-the-emergency-department/. Accessed June 2, 2023.

17. Akinosoglou K, Schinas G, Almyroudi MP, et al. The impact of age on intensive care. Ageing Res Rev 2023;84:101832.

Biofilm and Hospital-Acquired Infections in Older Adults

Patricia Stevenson, DNP, APRN, CNS-BC, CWS[a],*,
Melissa Marguet, DNP, MBA, RN[a],
Matthew Regulski, DPM, FFPM RCPS (Glasgow), ABMSP[a,b]

KEYWORDS

- Biofilm-associated disease • Critical care • Older adult
- Hospital-acquired infections • Treatment • Nursing care

KEY POINTS

- Biofilm infections are generally chronic in nature.
- Bacteria that reside within the biofilm structure are resilient against the immune system, antibiotics, and other traditional treatments.
- Prevention of hospital-acquired biofilm infections is the ultimate goal.
- To effectively treat biofilm infections, it is important to remove the protective biofilm structure.

INTRODUCTION

The complexities of biofilms and their impact on medically related infections are still being researched and are underestimated in direct care settings. Hoiby pointed out in a 2017 article that the aggregation of microbes that surrounded themselves with a self-produced matrix was described as early as 80 to 90 years ago.[1] However, it was not recognized as pathologic to human tissue until the late 1970s, when biofilm was isolated in the sputum of chronically infected cystic fibrosis patients.[1] By 1985, Costerton and colleagues had introduced the term biofilm and started the research avalanche, showing that biofilms increase quickly and are widespread in many disease states.[2] Research now supports that over 80% of all human infections are biofilm related, having 10 to 1000 times more resistance to antibiotics than previously realized.[3] Generally, tissue-related biofilm infections alter normal physiological organ function. They are frequently chronic, such as lung infections, osteomyelitis,

[a] Next Science™ LLC, 10550 Deerwood Park Boulevard, Suite 300, Jacksonville, FL 32256, USA;
[b] The Wound Institute of Ocean County, 54 Bey Lea Road Tom's River, NJ 08759, USA
* Corresponding author.
E-mail address: pstevenson@nextscience.com

Crit Care Nurs Clin N Am 35 (2023) 375–391
https://doi.org/10.1016/j.cnc.2023.05.007
0899-5885/23/© 2023 Elsevier Inc. All rights reserved.

prostatitis, rhinosinusitis, recurrent otitis media, urinary tract infections, endocarditis, periodontitis, and dental caries.[4] Biofilm can also be device-related, inhabiting tube insertion sites, residing on prosthetic devices, developing at hardware/pin exit sites, inhabiting chronic and surgical wounds, and have recently been identified in the altered microbiome of failing intact skin.[5–8] For older patients, the added exposure of living in institutional settings impacts possible exposure to higher-risk situations. In all cases, biofilm takes advantage of compromised innate immune defenses of older and debilitated patients and displays superior resistance to traditional infection treatments, including antibiotics.[9]

Biofilm is linked to the commonly discussed infections within the acute care setting known as hospital-acquired infections (HAIs). Older adults are at greater risk for HAI because of many factors, including immunosenescent cells, nutritional status, immobility issues, and an overall fragile state. The US Centers for Disease Control and Prevention (CDC) report roughly 687,000 infections to occur because of an HAI and estimate that the population over age 65 will double and those over 85 years will triple by 2060.[10–13] Roughly 3% of hospitalized patients have an HAI at a given time based on 2011 data. Urinary tract infections are the most common HAI (44% of all HAIs), with 57% attributed to *Escherichia coli*.[14] According to the CDC, HAI has an annual cost of over $28 billion.[11] Facing rising acuity and a growing population of older patients, HAI will continue to create more challenges to health care, requiring more treatments and services. Ongoing evide is providing clarity on biofilm's impact on HAI and the day-to-day care of patients in the intensive care unit (ICU), especially among the elderly.[9]

WHAT IS BIOFILM?

Biofilm is found in virtually every environment and begins as an aggregate of planktonic or free-swimming bacteria that attaches to objects, tissue, or devices and starts to accumulate (**Figs. 1** and **2**). Defined as a community of bacteria encased in a self-extruded exopolysaccharide matrix or protective slime, it continues to grow in a pathogenic life cycle if left undisturbed. Although matrix composition varies depending on

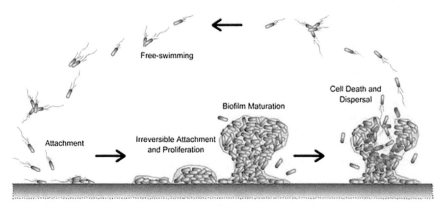

Fig. 1. Biofilm formation. (i) Attachment. Biofilm formation begins as an aggregate of bacteria that attaches to a surface or device. This phase is reversible. (ii) Growth. Bacteria form a protective barrier made of the EPS. The cells within proliferate, grow, and mature, creating an irreversible state. Quorum sensing occurs. (iii) Detachment. Part of the biofilm disperses and releases free-floating planktonic bacteria for further colonization. (Source: Barraud N. Nitric Oxide-Mediated Differentiation and Dispersal in Bacterial Biofilms. Thesis. UNSW Sydney; 2007. https://doi.org/10.26190/unsworks/17270.)

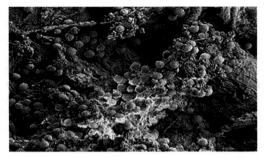

Fig. 2. Scanning electron micrograph (SEM) of *S aureus* biofilm growing in an in vitro wound model. Clusters of *S aureus* cells are coated by a stringy substance, thought to be EPS. It should be noted that during processing for SEM, the EPS becomes dehydrated and flattened. Image at X5, 000 magnification (Rumbaugh Laboratory) (Source: Rumbaugh, K. P. Biofilms in the ICU. The Southwest Respiratory and Critical Care Chronicles. 2014;2(6):15-18. https://doi.org/10.12746/swrccc2014.0206.067.)

the type of microbe and the growth environment, this protective slime layer generally comprises exopolysaccharides forming an extra polymeric substance (EPS), proteins, and extracellular DNA (eDNA) designed to shield the bacteria from external stressors.[15] Once the bacteria make the polysaccharide strands, metallic ion biosorption occurs from the environmental surroundings (iron, magnesium, zinc, and calcium). This provides the final element that strengthens the matrix and prevents the simple removal of biofilm, requiring targeted therapy to bind the metal ions, allowing the polysaccharide strands to return to a free-floating state. The EPS further facilitates the survival of the bacteria within the structure by blocking harmful molecules of antimicrobials, antibodies, and host inflammatory cells from reaching the bacteria, providing a diffusion barrier to small molecules such as antibiotics so they fail to reach the encased bacteria.[16,17] As a result of this survival instinct, the EPS can be triggered to increase rapidly in the case of disruption, fragmenting, or assault, causing biofilm to reform more quickly.[18]

Bacteria encased within the biofilm differ from planktonic or free-swimming bacteria in several ways. Planktonic bacteria are unable to withstand the direct assault from antimicrobials, antiseptics, or disinfectants that have been traditionally used to combat bacterial infections. However, bacteria within a biofilm exhibit a sophisticated relationship of cooperative protective effects through RNA and DNA transfer, share a reduced susceptibility to antibiotics, and exhibit dormancy to avoid immune detection.[16,17,19]

Biofilm Origination and Formation

Biofilm originates from exogenous or endogenous bacterial inoculation via community or healthcare-associated exposures.[20] **Fig. 1** depicts how bacteria attach and form the EPS matrix, which varies in minutes to hours and among bacterial phenotypes such as *E coli*, methicillin-resistant *Staphylococcus aureus* (MRSA), and *Pseudomonas aeruginosa*. All research indicates the stages of a biofilm life cycle are consistent regardless of exposure and type of surface attachment. The biofilm-producing bacteria can attach in minutes, form an irreversible attachment within 2 to 4 hours, form the protective EPS structure, and become tolerant of antibiotics and antiseptics within 6 to 12 hours (for bacteria within the structure). This process is much faster than previously believed, with recovery from disruption often occurring within 24 hours.[21]

Once bacteria attach and begin to form the matrix, the consequences to clinical practice become more profound. During the life cycle stages (see **Fig. 1**), the biofilm continues to expand until the final stage, when new bacteria or microcolonies of clustered biofilm burst from the established colonies and recolonize in new areas. When this happens, and the bacteria travel through the bloodstream, seeding can occur and produce diverse infections, severely affecting patients, and grow undetected until the biofilm interferes with normal function. Because of the ability of the biofilm infection to exhibit subclinical signs and symptoms, patients often are severely sick before the infections are recognized, as in the case of endocarditis with biofilm vegetation.[22]

Biofilm Eradication

After matrix formation, biofilm cannot be easily removed even in cases of surgical debridement without biofilm-targeted interventions and specifically interventions that solubilize the protective structure. Gloag and colleagues identified that shearing and chemical assault on biofilm stimulates the EPS to form more biofilm reserves, as depicted in (**Fig. 3**).[23] Unfortunately, internal biofilm infections are difficult, if not impossible, to eradicate.

Between growth cycles, new outbreaks of facultative human pathogens can form biofilms outside the body and survive and maintain a high infectious dose for prolonged periods. One example has been observed with hospital-acquired outbreaks of *Candida auris* pathogens that can live on disinfected surfaces and represent a hazard for future infections.[19] Suggested strategies to combat biofilm include preventing the initial attachment, minimizing the biofilm formation, and targeting the EPS structure.[24]

HOW BIOFILMS INFLUENCE DISEASE STATES

Until confocal laser scanning microscopy (CLSM) became available in 1957, the medical community believed all bacteria responded to antibiotic therapy or topical

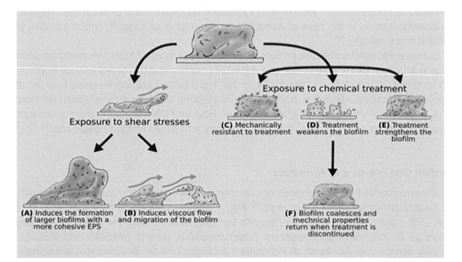

Fig. 3. Schematic of how biofilm mechanics can influence survival. Summary of how biofilm viscoelasticity can protect the microbial community when exposed to (*A, B*) mechanical forces, such as shear stress, and (*C–F*) chemical treatment. (Source: Gloag ES, Fabbri S, Wozniak DJ, Stoodley P. Biofilm mechanics: Implications in infection and survival. Biofilm. 2020;2:100017. https://doi.org/10.1016/j.bioflm.2019.100017.)

antiseptics.[25] Still, as further sophisticated testing evolved, the discovery of biofilm's recalcitrant and tolerant nature has been observed, especially in several disease states connected to biofilm (**Fig. 4**). It may be considered a primary or secondary biofilm infection (**Fig. 5**). For example, recently, biofilm was discovered within ruptured vertebral discs, cases of dry eye, and asymptomatic bacteriuria.[26–28] Biofilm formation is a common feature in human pathology. Because of its microscopic size, no point-of-care test is available to detect biofilm.

Recalcitrant Nature of Biofilm

Biofilm is linked to the commonly discussed infections within the hospital environment, including critical care, known as HAIs. These include surgical site infections (SSI), ventilator-associated pneumonia (VAP), central line-associated bloodstream infection (CLABSI), and catheter-associated urinary tract infection (CAUTI). HAIs are more prominent in the aging population, especially in long-term care and skilled nursing facilities. They are predisposed because of the need for indwelling devices and typically

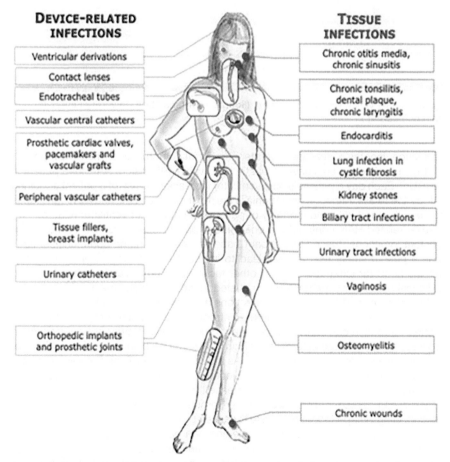

DEVICE-RELATED INFECTIONS

- Ventricular derivations
- Contact lenses
- Endotracheal tubes
- Vascular central catheters
- Prosthetic cardiac valves, pacemakers and vascular grafts
- Peripheral vascular catheters
- Tissue fillers, breast implants
- Urinary catheters
- Orthopedic implants and prosthetic joints

TISSUE INFECTIONS

- Chronic otitis media, chronic sinusitis
- Chronic tonsilitis, dental plaque, chronic laryngitis
- Endocarditis
- Lung infection in cystic fibrosis
- Kidney stones
- Biliary tract infections
- Urinary tract infections
- Vaginosis
- Osteomyelitis
- Chronic wounds

Fig. 4. Biofilm-associated infections. (Source: Høiby N, Bjarnsholt T, Moser C, et al. ESCMID* guideline for the diagnosis and treatment of biofilm infections 2014. Clinical Microbiology and Infection. 2015;21:S1-S25. https://doi.org/10.1016/j.cmi.2014.10.024.)

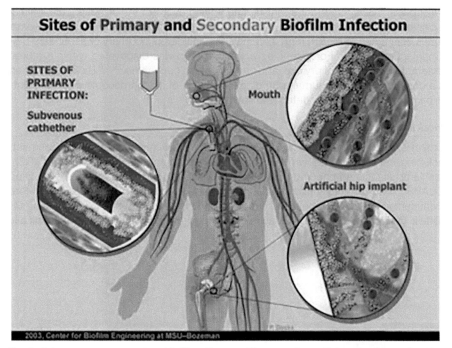

Fig. 5. Primary versus secondary biofilm. (Source: Montana State University Center for Biofilm Engineering.)

have longer lengths of stay and a greater number of comorbidities. The CDC reports 1 in 31 hospitalized patients have at least 1 HAI, with a 19% risk of HAIs for a patient in the ICU.[10] Each day a patient is on a ventilator increases the risk of a patient acquiring VAP by 1% to 3%. Although pneumonia is the most common HAI, and although it does increase the morbidity and mortality of patients, most are not ventilator related.[13] In-hospital-related HAIs contribute to one-third of patient deaths. Linked to multidrug-resistant infections, these HAIs impact patients and their home communities. HAIs pose a patient safety risk, as they lead to increased antibiotic use, length of stay, and the need for extended stays at other facilities for rehabilitation, often requiring additional procedures, primarily when related to wound development.[29,30]

Many device- and tissue-related infections are attributable to biofilm, as shown in (**Figs. 4-6**). Like any invasive procedure, introducing a catheter, urinary catheter, or tracheal intubation can introduce bacteria through the skin barrier or via introduction into a sterile site through external openings.[24] A Saudi Arabian study showed 20% of pressure injuries were device-related.[31] As indicated by **Fig. 7**, biofilm can be inoculated by inserting catheters, devices, or injections, essentially dragging bacteria into a new site, which facilitates bacteria to increase through the biofilm life cycle.[24]

Biofilm can spread in many ways, either through direct external inoculation or by seeding. Gingivitis/periodontal disease is caused by biofilm that forms between cleanings. Internally, bacterial and biofilm seeding can occur from a previous infection, dental caries, or mature dental plaque and sometimes occur with dental cleanings when bleeding during the procedure inoculates the bloodstream (**Fig. 8**).[32] Additionally, older patients often have poor oral status from worsened physical conditions, a lack of regular dental care, and cumulative damage caused by dental diseases in

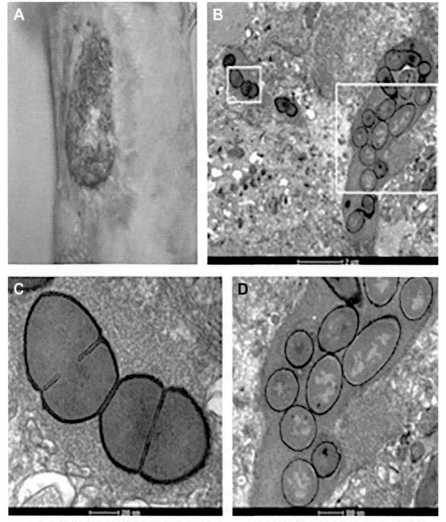

Fig. 6. Bacterial biofilm in chronic venous ulcer. (*A*) Venous leg ulcer of a 33-year-old woman with a history of deep vein thrombosis in the left leg and pulmonary embolism. This wound was present in left medial malleolus for 2 years, showing 15.37 cm² and 40% of yellow necrotic tissue. (*B*) Bacterial colonies showing spherical and rod-shaped cells seen by transmission electron microscopy. (*C, D*) Bacteria surrounded by a dense extracellular matrix. (Source: Honorato-Sampaio K, Martins Guedes AC, Nogueira Lima VLDA, Borges EL. Bacterial biofilm in chronic venous ulcer. The Brazilian Journal of Infectious Diseases. 2014;18(3):350-351. https://doi.org/10.1016/j.bjid.2014.01.003.)

the past.[33] These diseases can also lead to systemic inflammation and other more serious complication such as pericarditis.[22]

HOW BIOFILM IMPACTS THE CRITICAL ELDERLY

Identifying infection in the critically ill before it reaches a stage where it is life-threatening is challenging. It requires improved awareness on the part of caregivers,

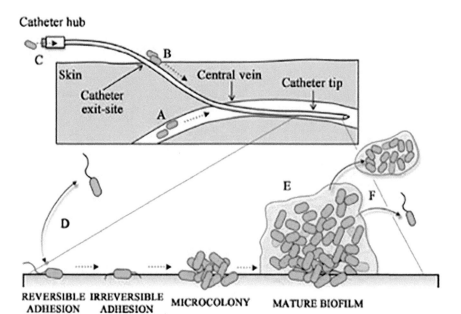

Fig. 7. Biofilm formation during catheterization. (Source: Kabir CMdN. Catheter induced urinary tract infection: post-surgical prevalence with curative and preventive management. OALib. 2022;09(12):1-11. https://doi.org/10.4236/oalib.1109513.)

focused monitoring of at-risk patients, and extra care when performing high-risk procedures (**Fig. 9**). Biofilm is initially not visible and generally requires more intuitive recognition of signs or symptoms that a biofilm may be present. The biofilm can manifest as wound slough and fibrin, drainage color and consistency changes, and recurring infections despite treatment with antibiotics or standard therapies.[34] Historically, unresolved infection was termed critical colonization, a phrase associated with impending acute infection, but biofilm-associated infections can be more dangerous than a high level of bacteria.

When the biofilm is present, the immune response is blunted and subverted by the biofilm life cycle. Inflammation and the aging immune system prevent older ICU patients from mounting a robust response to bacterial invasion before actual attachment, allowing the transition from planktonic to a biofilm state of attached bacteria. Cells age as people get older. In older patients, cell turnover or apoptosis (programmed cellular death) slows and allows these older cells to promote constant low levels of inflammatory factors, the cornerstone of human disease and infection, which further augments

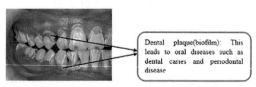

Fig. 8. Dental Plaque-Oral Biofilm. (Source: Abebe GM. Oral biofilm and its impact on oral health, psychological and social interaction. Int J Oral Dent Health. 2021;7(1). https://doi. org/10.23937/2469-5734/1510127.)

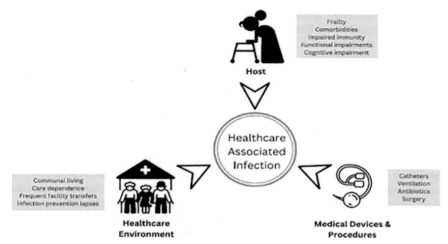

Fig. 9. Medical treatments, host, and environmental factors all contribute to the increased susceptibility of healthcare-associated infections in older adults. (Source: Tesini BL, Dumyati G. Healthcare-associated infections in older adults: epidemiology and prevention. Infect Dis Clin North Am. 2023;37(1):65-86. https://doi.org/10.1016/j.idc.2022.11.004.)

the disease state and contributes to the difficulty in identifying a biofilm infection **Box 1**.

Biofilm-associated infections may initially respond to antibiotic therapy by reducing the numbers of planktonic bacteria; however, cardinal signs and symptoms of biofilm will present as the biofilm increases. For example, when a patient fails to progress through a normal and timely healing sequence exhibiting prolonged inflammation, waxing and waning of symptoms only to return as if untreated through persistent or recurrent infections or displays an overall failure to improve, he or she likely has biofilm.[35] Often this failure to improve is in tandem with overarching comorbid conditions that conceal the underlying biofilm infection. Elderly immune systems are compromised, even without infection, and laboratory results may show continuously stimulated immune cells that superficially may be attributed to other conditions while a biofilm may be thriving.

Box 1
Main risk factors of biofilm infections in older intensive care unit patients

- Admission to ICU and need for invasive procedures.
- Aging immune system (immunosenescent)
- Comorbid conditions
- Prolonged hospitalization
- Previous exposure to HAI infections or history of previous infection
- Foreign bodies (central lines, intravenous lines, indwelling catheters), mechanical ventilation.
- Open wounds and pressure injuries
- Fresh surgical sites
- Incontinence

Bioburden reduction primarily relies on nurses to apply a holistic biofilm-aware approach to patient care through thorough biofilm-focused assessments not relying on testing to determine if a biofilm may be present.[34,36–39] Biofilms are not visible and practically undetectable. Currently, standard bedside wound cultures can only identify pathogens outside of a biofilm, while bacteria within a biofilm remain viable but nonculturable (VBNC)[40] Because biofilm-encased bacteria are VBNC, many sites have implemented more sophisticated analysis methods such as next-generation sequencing (NGS) with polymerase chain reaction (PCR) amplification, which can identify bacteria within a biofilm.[37] However, not all facilities have this testing available.

A negative culture of a surface or wound does not indicate that biofilm is absent, as the bacteria encased within a biofilm cannot be reached to culture. Despite biofilm's ubiquitous nature, there are strategies nursing can implement at the bedside to aid in the prevention and reduce the proliferation of biofilm. One strategy directly targets the biofilm structure. Utilizing agents that penetrate and remove the biofilm EPS structure to facilitate reaching and destroying the bacterial cells within is optimal for aiding biofilm removal.[39] For areas that can be reached, selective sharp debridement is suggested as the first-line method for removing bioburden from the site; however, consideration for the biofilm's presence beyond the necrotic and contaminated tissue or hardware should be made. Often, debridement alone cannot eliminate biofilm within a site, and the proliferation of the biofilm will continue. Choosing agents specifically designed to target the biofilm structure, such as those that can bind the metallic ions that hold the biofilm structure together, should be considered.

Another strategy nurses can implement is to eliminate cell-to-cell communication among planktonic bacteria by using bactericidal agents that kill the free-swimming bacteria before they can form a biofilm.[41] Dressing and antimicrobial agents are available that target the free-swimming and dispersed bacteria at the beginning and final stages of the biofilm life cycle but may have a limited impact on the biofilm structure (**Table 1**).[39] Products to utilize should, by nature, be broad spectrum, biocompatible with host tissue, protect the wound from infections and microorganisms, and decrease surface necrosis[42] The process of bioburden reduction also requires a holistic nursing approach to help boost the patient's immune system, such as augmenting the patient's nutritional status, advocating for treatments that target the biofilm structure, and using proper techniques when performing invasive procedures.

Biofilm Prevention at the Bedside

Critical care nurses play a vital role in infection prevention, as they are typically the first to assess and manage the patient and determine if an infection is developing. Highly trained nurses, aware of biofilms and the risks of HAI, can help reduce the spread of infections, including biofilms. Recognizing that the older adult in critical care has a high risk for acquiring an HAI, exceptional individualized care is essential to identify causative microorganisms and prevent or decrease the incidence and spread of these preventable infections. **Fig. 10** depicts the biofilm activities and specific moments where the biofilm and its cells and structure are most vulnerable to eradication.[36]

CLINIC CARE POINTS

There are some basic nursing strategies that should occur to aid in reducing biofilm-related infections (**Fig. 11**).

The simplest way to effectively prevent infections is by practicing hand hygiene. The CDC lists washing hands with soap and water or using alcohol-based hand sanitizer as the primary method to prevent the spread of infection.[43] Eye care to avoid dry

Table 1
Biofilm target strategies

Goal: Target EPS Structure and Break Down the Metallic Bonds Holding Structure Together, Prevent the Biofilm Pathogens from Recolonizing.	
Strategy	**Current Treatment Options**
Antimicrobials	• Cannot dismantle the biofilm structure • Nonselective and can impact both host cells and pathogens • At effective strengths maybe cytotoxic, often with the EPS depleting the reactive agents prior to getting to the pathogens • Unable to fully penetrate biofilm and may only kill active bacteria on the surface.
Antibiotics	• Broad-spectrum antimicrobial with variable tissue compatibility • Cannot dismantle the biofilm structure with little utility against biofilm. Effectiveness decreases and has been connected to antimicrobial resistance.
Outpatient sharp debridement	• Nonselective with no microbial resistance • Does not have sustained biofilm barrier impact • Pathogens left behind will recolonize
Dispersing agents	• Dissolve biofilm and cause microbial lysis • Are broad spectrum and do not promote microbial resistance • Compatible with tissue and provide a sustained biofilm barrier

Wolcott, R. (2015). Disrupting the biofilm matrix improves wound healing outcomes. Journal of Wound Care 24(8), 366-71. https://doi.org/10.12968/jowc.2015.24.8.366; and Kim, P.A. (2018, February 23). Clinic-based debridement of chronic ulcers has minimal impact on bacteria. Retrieved from Wounds 30(5) 114-119; and Snyder, R. B. (et al) (2017). Wound Biofilm: current perspectives and strategies on biofilm disruption and treatments. Wounds Supplement 29(6 suppl), S1-S17.

eyes (now viewed as induced by biofilm), oral care, and meticulous care of preferential biofilm growth sites such as the axilla and perineal areas must be stressed as important nursing tasks. Among all patients, the warm, moist, and nutrient-rich oral cavity is considered an incubator for diverse microbial species in their planktonic and sessile states. The patient's oral health can serve as an indicator of the patient's overall health and well-being. Careful attention to these areas is a first line of defense against the internal spread of biofilm.

Catheters and Devices

There are specific prevention strategies nurses can implement to prevent a CAUTI infection in addition to standard precautions. For example, inserting catheters only when indicated and remove when no longer needed. Nurses should follow proper techniques during insertion and maintenance and practice hand hygiene before and after contact with a patient, the surroundings, and catheter components—maintenance of a closed drainage system, unobstructed urine flow, and keeping a drainage bag below the bladder. The most common pathogen for a CAUTI is E coli, from fecal contamination. Therefore, perform perineal and periurethral care at least daily or, when indicated, treating, and addressing skin folds that can harbor bacteria.[24]

Vascular Access Devices

Central line insertion and management should include sterile practices routinely.[44] The insertion site should be inspected daily or per facility policies to assess for possible

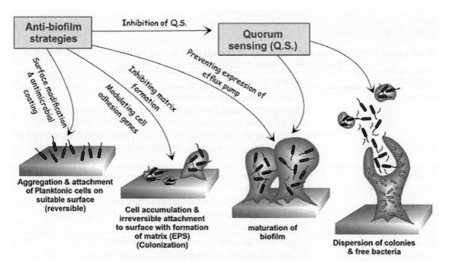

Fig. 10. The stages of biofilm formation and potential targets for anti-biofilm agents. The bacterial cells in people attach to the matrix-forming proteins by forming a covalent linkage with peptidoglycan structure or by noncovalent attachment. With attachment and aggregation of a sufficient number of cells, the formation of EPS matrix takes place, and the attachment now becomes resistant to external repulsive forces. With the maturation of biofilm, the cells within the bulk structure start further communication with each other and start secreting specialized proteins and DNA, and some of them are involved in the formation of the efflux pump. At last, the dispersion of free planktonic cells from the formed biofilm further promotes the formation of new biofilms in the periphery. The natural anti-biofilm compounds can attack at one or different stages of biofilm formation and development, thus inhibiting it. (Source: Mishra R, Panda AK, De Mandal S, Shakeel M, Bisht SS, Khan J. Natural anti-biofilm agents: strategies to control biofilm-forming pathogens. Front Microbiol. 2020;11:566325. https://doi.org/10.3389/fmicb.2020.566325.)

infection and proper functioning. Following hospital protocol that requires disinfecting ports, connectors, and hubs will help prevent the spread of infection. Sterile technique should be strictly followed during dressing changes. Dressing changes should occur every 5 to 7 days or when the dressing seal is broken, the dressing is visibly soiled, or per facility policy.

Oral Care

The oral flora has been directly linked to infections such as hospital-acquired pneumonia and in sternal incisions after cardiac surgery. By providing regular oral care, the natural microbiome of the oral cavity can be restored and help prevent biofilm growth.[12] Increased biofilm pathogenic colonization is a result of poor dentition. Ensuring oral hygiene can help minimize the risk of a patient developing a secondary infection. Oral hygiene should include brushing the teeth, cleansing the gums if no teeth are present, and inspecting the oral cavity if on a ventilator, as this patient population is at a greater risk of aspiration and respiratory infections.

Wound Care

Prevention and the care of wounds in older adults are essential. Comorbid conditions, immobility, and a failing skin barrier can predispose older patients to skin breakdown

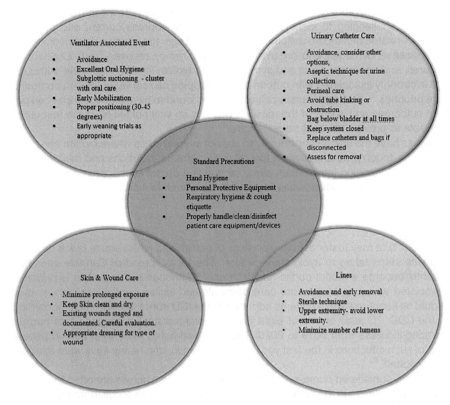

Fig. 11. Main risk factors of biofilm infection in older patients.

and the development of wound-related biofilm. Wounds on patients in the ICU should be covered with an appropriate dressing at all times and receive dressing changes as indicated by the wound characteristics, such as drainage. Frequent nursing assessments and preventative measures should be in place to avoid new pressure injuries and provide optimal healing of existing wounds.[31]

DISCUSSION

According to the National Center for Health Statistics, life expectancy in the United States fell in 2021 to just over 76 years of age. Still, according to a 2020 article in *Critical Care*, Hass and colleagues found that older patients (defined as $\geq$ 70 years old) have a higher risk of death and functional decline than younger patients, with age as a proxy representing the likelihood of survival.[45,46]

Currently, the median age of critically ill patients approaches 65 years, with the proportion of the very old ($\geq$ 80 years of age) on the rise.[9] As the population ages, an increasing proportion of critical care admissions will be the elderly with physical and functional body alterations, predisposing them to infections. Older patients are often immunocompromised with low and failing immune responses, senescent cellular activity, and continuous levels of inflammation from comorbid conditions that factor into daily nursing care.[9] Additionally, comorbid conditions associated with aging compound the degradation of cellular responses and exacerbate inflammatory states, making it challenging to identify care pathways that address current and potential infection-related healthcare deficits. With increased age, the additive risks of diabetes, heart disease, dementia, end-organ failure, polypharmacy, recovery from surgical procedures, and obscured signs and symptoms of a biofilm infection increase. Although age is strongly associated with outcomes, overlapping clinical variables can confound care priorities.[47,48] Missed nursing care has been found to have a direct impact on patient outcomes and is one of the reasons why it is so vital nurses have the resources available to provide the best bedside care.[49–51]

Nurses have the unique opportunity to impact several areas where biofilm can manifest. High-touch procedures such as oral care, catheter insertions and maintenance, initiating or changing intravenous sites, central line dressing changes, and endotracheal tube care are opportunities to prevent a biofilm infection.

SUMMARY

Situations that may foster the development of biofilm and HAIs require quick recognition with steps taken to avoid transmission. The rapid spread of *Candida auris* has recently become a global public health threat.[49] Although the organism is primarily associated with long-term acute care hospitals and skilled nursing facilities, nurses should be keenly aware of patients admitted to the ICU from these facilities. According to the CDC, "*C auris* is one of eight antimicrobial-resistant pathogens that had an alarming increase from 2019 to 2020. The CDC estimated more than 29,400 people died of such infections in the first year of the pandemic, and nearly 40% were infected in a hospital".[49]

HAIs are considered nurse-sensitive outcomes because nurses are often the first to recognize a change in the patient's status.[52] Although it takes a collaborative team to address HAIs, the bedside nurse has the most significant responsibility and duty to implement evidence-based practices to address biofilm-related infections. This is especially important in the older population at the most significant risk for developing or acquiring an HAI. Biofilm is not going away. As nurses become more familiar with biofilm and how it impacts their patients, patients will benefit from the creative practices nurses can bring to the ICU. Changes in bedside practice are quality puzzles that nurses can solve through procedural adjustments and the establishment of best practices.

DISCLOSURE

P. Stevenson is a paid clinical consultant of Next Science, LLC, and M. Marguet is a paid employee of Next Science, LLC, 10,550 Deerwood Park Boulevard, Suite 300, Jacksonville, FL 32256. Dr M. Regulski is the Medical Director for Next Science, LLC and served as subject matter expert. No funding was provided for this project.

REFERENCES

1. Høiby N, Bjarnsholt T, Moser C, et al. ESCMID* guideline for the diagnosis and treatment of biofilm infections 2014. Clin Microbiol Infection 2015;21:S1–25. https://doi.org/10.1016/j.cmi.2014.10.024.

2. Costerton JW, Lewandowski Z, Caldwell DE, et al. Microbial biofilms. Annu Rev Microbiol 1995;49:711–45. https://doi.org/10.1146/annurev.mi.49.100195.003431.

3. Sharma D, Misba L, Khan AU. Antibiotics versus biofilm: an emerging battle-ground in microbial communities. Antimicrob Resist Infect Control 2019;8:76. https://doi.org/10.1186/s13756-019-0533-3.

4. Burmølle M, Thomsen TR, Fazli M, et al. Biofilms in chronic infections–a matter of opportunity–monospecies biofilms in multispecies infections. FEMS Immunol Med Microbiol 2010;59(3):324–36. https://doi.org/10.1111/j.1574-695X.2010. 00714.x.

5. Donlan RM, Costerton JW. Biofilms: survival mechanisms of clinically relevant microorganisms. Clin Microbiol Rev 2002;15(2):167–93. https://doi.org/10.1128/ CMR.15.2.167-193.2002.

6. Parsek MR, Singh PK. Bacterial biofilms: an emerging link to disease pathogenesis. Annu Rev Microbiol 2003;57:677–701. https://doi.org/10.1146/annurev. micro.57.030502.090720.

7. Metcalf DG, Bowler PG. Biofilm delays wound healing: a review of the evidence. Burns Trauma 2013;1(1):5–12. https://doi.org/10.4103/2321-3868.113329.

8. Brandwein M, Steinberg D, Meshner S. Microbial biofilms and the human skin microbiome. npj Biofilms Microbiomes 2016;2(1):3. https://doi.org/10.1038/s41522-016-0004-z.

9. Esme M, Topeli A, Yavuz BB, et al. Infections in the elderly critically ill patients. Front Med 2019;6:118. https://doi.org/10.3389/fmed.2019.00118.

10. Hai data | CDC. Published March 3, 2023. Available at: https://www.cdc.gov/hai/ data/index.html. Accessed March 30, 2023.

11. Centers for Disease Control and Prevention (CDC). Office of the Associate Director for Policy and Strategy. Healthcare-associated infections (HAI). Last reviewed June 21, 2021. Available at: https://www.cdc.gov/hai/index.html. Accessed February 5, 2023.

12. Centers for Disease Control and Prevention (CDC), National Center for Emerging and Zoonotic Infectious Diseases (NCEZID), Division of Healthcare Quality Promotion (DHQP). Updated November 3, 2022. Available at: https://www.cdc. gov/hai/data/portal/index.html. Accessed February 20, 2023.

13. Tesini BL, Dumyati G. Health care-associated infections in older adults: epidemiology and prevention. Infect Dis Clin North Am 2023;37(1):65–86. https://doi.org/ 10.1016/j.idc.2022.11.004.

14. Maharjan G, Khadka P, Siddhi Shilpakar G, et al. Catheter-associated urinary tract infection and obstinate biofilm producers. Can J Infect Dis Med Microbiol 2018;2018:1–7. https://doi.org/10.1155/2018/7624857.

15. Flemming HC, Wingender J. The biofilm matrix. Nat Rev Microbiol 2010;8(9): 623–33. https://doi.org/10.1038/nrmicro2415.

16. Hall-Stoodley L, Stoodley P. Evolving concepts in biofilm infections. Cell Microbiol 2009;11(7):1034–43. https://doi.org/10.1111/j.1462-5822.2009.01323.x.

17. Brooun A, Liu S, Lewis K. A dose-response study of antibiotic resistance in pseudomonas aeruginosa biofilms. Antimicrob Agents Chemother 2000;44(3):640-646. Available at: https://www.ncbi.nlm.nih.gov/pmc/articles/PMC89739/. Accessed March 30, 2023.

18. Tseng BS, Reichhardt C, Merrihew GE, et al. A biofilm matrix-associated protease inhibitor protects pseudomonas aeruginosa from proteolytic attack. mBio 2018; 9(2). https://doi.org/10.1128/mBio.00543-18. e00543-18.

19. Schulze A, Mitterer F, Pombo JP, et al. Biofilms by bacterial human pathogens: clinical relevance-development, composition and regulation-therapeutical strategies. Microb Cell 2021;8(2):28–56. https://doi.org/10.15698/mic2021.02.741.

20. Liu S, Lu H, Zhang S, et al. Phages against pathogenic bacterial biofilms and biofilm-based infections: a review. Pharmaceutics 2022;14(2):427. https://doi.org/10.3390/pharmaceutics14020427.

21. Katsuyama M, Ichikawa H, Ogawa S, et al. A novel method to control the balance of skin microflora. Part 1. Attack on biofilm of *Staphylococcus aureus* without antibiotics. J Dermatol Sci 2005;38(3):197–205. https://doi.org/10.1016/j.jdermsci.2005.01.006 [published correction appears in J Dermatol Sci. 2005 Sep;39(3):196. Masako, Katsuyama [corrected to Katsuyama, Masako]; Hideyuki, Ichikawa [corrected to Ichikawa, Hideyuki]; Shigeyuki, Ogawa [corrected to Ogawa, Shigeyuki]; Zenro, Ikezawa [corrected to Ikezawa, Zenro]].

22. Lerche CJ, Schwartz F, Theut M, et al. Anti-biofilm approach in infective endocarditis exposes new treatment strategies for improved outcome. Front Cell Dev Biol 2021;9:643335. doi:10.3389/fcell.2021.643335.

23. Gloag ES, Fabbri S, Wozniak DJ, et al. Biofilm mechanics: implications in infection and survival. Biofilm 2020;2:100017. https://doi.org/10.1016/j.bioflm.2019.100017.

24. Lindsay D, von Holy A. Bacterial biofilms within the clinical setting: what healthcare professionals should know. J Hosp Infect 2006;64(4):313–25. https://doi.org/10.1016/j.jhin.2006.06.028.

25. Kihm KD. Chapter 4: Confocal laser scanning microscopy (CLSM), In: Tropea C, Rival D, Near-field characterization of micro/nano-scaled fluid flows. Experimental fluid mechanics, 2011, Springer; Berlin, 55-79. doi:10.1007/978-3-642-20426-5_4.

26. Senker W, Aspalter S, Radl C, et al. Frequency and characteristics of bacterial and viral low-grade infections of the intervertebral discs: a prospective, observational study. J Orthop Traumatol 2022;23(1):15. https://doi.org/10.1186/s10195-022-00633-y.

27. Vincent M, Quintero J, D. Perry H, et al. Biofilm theory for lid margin and dry eye disease. In: Kopacz D, ed. Ocular surface diseases-some current date on tear film problem and keratoconic diagnosis. IntechOpen 2021;63(2):257-269.

28. Mouton C, Bazaldua O, Pierce B, et al. Common infections in older adults. Am Fam Physician 2001;63(2):257–69.

29. Rogers AE. Chapter 40: The Effects of Fatigue and Sleepiness on Nurse Performance and Patient Safety. In: Hughes RG. editor. Patient Safety and Quality: An Evidence-Based Handbook for Nurses. Rockville (MD): Agency for Healthcare Research and Quality (US); 2008, 2-509 - 2-545. Available at: https://www.ncbi.nlm.nih.gov/books/NBK2645/.

30. Haque M, Sartelli M, McKimm J, et al. Health care-associated infections-an overview. Infect Drug Resist 2018;11:2321–33.

31. Al-Dorzi H. Prevention of pressure injury in the intensive care unit. Saudi Crit Care J 2019;3(1):24. https://doi.org/10.4103/2543-1854.259474.

32. Chhaliyil P, Fischer K, Schoel B, et al. A novel, simple, frequent oral cleaning method reduces damaging bacteria in the dental microbiota. J Int Soc Prevent Communit Dent 2020;10(4):511. https://doi.org/10.4103/jispcd.JISPCD_31_20.

33. Leung KC, Chu CH. Dental care for older adults. Int J Environ Res Public Health 2022;20(1):214.

34. Schultz G, Bjarnsholt T, James GA, et al. Consensus guidelines for the identification and treatment of biofilms in chronic nonhealing wounds: guidelines for chronic wound biofilms. Wound Rep and Reg 2017;25(5):744–57. https://doi.org/10.1111/wrr.12590.

35. Attinger C, Wolcott R. Clinically addressing biofilm in chronic wounds. Adv Wound Care 2012;1(3):127–32. https://doi.org/10.1089/wound.2011.0333.
36. Mishra R, Panda AK, De Mandal S, et al. Natural anti-biofilm agents: strategies to control biofilm-forming pathogens. Front Microbiol 2020;11:566325. https://doi.org/10.3389/fmicb.2020.566325.
37. Baldan R, Se P. Precision medicine in the diagnosis and management of orthopedic biofilm infections. Front Med 2020;7:580671. https://doi.org/10.3389/fmed.2020.580671.
38. Rumbaugh KP. Biofilms in the ICU. SWRCCC 2014;2(6). https://doi.org/10.12746/swrccc2014.0206.067.
39. Phillips PL, Wolcott RD, Fletcher J, et al. Biofilms made easy. Wounds International 2010;1(3).1-6. Available at: https://www.woundsinternational.com/resources/details/biofilms-made-easy. Accessed March 30, 2023.
40. Trevors JT. Viable but non-culturable (VBNC) bacteria: gene expression in planktonic and biofilm cells. J Microbiol Methods 2011;86(2):266–73. https://doi.org/10.1016/j.mimet.2011.04.018.
41. Davies DG, Parsek MR, Pearson JP, et al. The involvement of cell-to-cell signals in the development of a bacterial biofilm. Science 1998;280(5361):295–8.
42. Rezvani Ghomi E, Khalili S, Nouri Khorasani S, et al. Wound dressings: current advances and future directions. J Appl Polym Sci 2019;136:47738.
43. Centers for Disease Control and Prevention. Hand hygiene in healthcare settings | handwashing |. Published July 28, 2022. Available at: https://www.cdc.gov/handwashing/handwashing-healthcare.html. Accessed March 30, 2023.
44. Hicks MA, Lopez PP. Central line management. In: StatPearls. StatPearls Publishing; 2023. Available at: http://www.ncbi.nlm.nih.gov/books/NBK539811/. Accessed March 30, 2023.
45. Arias E, Tejada-Vera B, Kochanek K, et al. Provisional life expectancy estimates for 2021. Vital Statistics Rapid Release. Report 23. Published August 2022. Available at: https://www.cdc.gov/nchs/data/vsrr/vsrr023.pdf. Accessed March 20, 2023.
46. Haas LEM, De Lange DW, Van Dijk D, et al. Should we deny ICU admission to the elderly? Ethical considerations in times of COVID-19. Crit Care 2020;24(1):321. https://doi.org/10.1186/s13054-020-03050-x.
47. Vosylius S. Determinants of outcome in elderly patients admitted to the intensive care unit. Age Ageing 2005;34(2):157–62. https://doi.org/10.1093/ageing/afi037.
48. CDC. Covid-19 & antibiotic resistance. Centers for Disease Control and Prevention. Published August 11, 2022. Available at: https://www.cdc.gov/drugresistance/covid19.htmL. Accessed March 30, 2023.
49. Mynaříková E, Jarošová D, Janíková E, et al. Occurrence of hospital-acquired infections in relation to missed nursing care: a literature review. Cent Eur J Nurs Midw 2020;11(1):43–9. https://doi.org/10.15452/cejnm.2020.11.0007.
50. Kalisch BJ, Xie B. Errors of omission: missed nursing care. West J Nurs Res 2014;36(7):875–90. https://doi.org/10.1177/0193945914531859.
51. Marguet MA, Ogaz V. The effect of a teamwork intervention on staff perception of teamwork and patient care on a medical surgical unit. Nurs Forum 2019;54(2):171–82. https://doi.org/10.1111/nuf.12311.
52. Boev C, Kiss E. Hospital-acquired infections. Crit Care Nurs Clin 2017;29(1):51–65. https://doi.org/10.1016/j.cnc.2016.09.012.

Progressive Supranuclear Palsy

Challenges and Considerations for Care Transitions

Nadine Wodwaski, DNP, MSN-ed, CNS, RN

KEYWORDS

- Progressive supranuclear palsy • Nursing • Clinical nurse specialist • Care transition

KEY POINTS

- Progressive supranuclear palsy (PSP) is a fatal neurological disease that presents as disequilibrium, unsteadiness, dizziness with unexplained falls and supranuclear gaze.
- Many PSP patient will be admitted to the intensive care unit due to fall injuries, choking or aspiration pneumonia.
- The aim of nursing care should reflect life maintenance.
- Patients with PSP undergoing care transition are at an increased risk of undesirable clinical outcomes such as, ICU-acquired skeletal muscle mass wasting, post-ICU mind, body, and emotional symptoms, and morbidity and mortality due to frequently poor communication and inconsistent care.
- Through the 3 spheres of impact, Clinical Nurse Specialists can educate, support and guide patients with PSP /families, aiding in the successful care transition.

PROGRESSIVE SUPRANUCLEAR PALSY: CHALLENGES AND CONSIDERATIONS FOR CARE TRANSITIONS

Nurses are the most trusted profession globally,[1] thanks to the provisional and coordinated patient care, education, and compassion they provide to patients, families, and communities. Nurses genuinely listen to the needs, fears, concerns, thoughts, and feelings of others. Respectively, nursing encompasses an art, a belief that individuals have value.

Nurses practice with an innate sense of ethical tenets and possess a keen sense of knowing when to take action. They have the opportunity to heal their patients' hearts,

There are no financial conflicts of interest to disclose.
University of Detroit Mercy, 4001 West McNichols Road, Detroit, MI 48221, USA
E-mail address: wodwasnk@udmercy.edu

Crit Care Nurs Clin N Am 35 (2023) 393–401
https://doi.org/10.1016/j.cnc.2023.05.008
0899-5885/23/© 2023 Elsevier Inc. All rights reserved.

minds, and souls. As a result of these proficiencies, nurses are integral members of the health care team coordinating, managing, and caring for distinct and challenging patients. With their frontline expertise and contribution to care, the linchpin of health care continues.

Throughout many nursing careers, professional nurses contribute to society, constantly meeting the health care needs of patients from birth to death. It is a gift. When patients with a terminal illness are admitted to the health care organization, nurses can help patients through this challenging time. One such illness is progressive supranuclear palsy (PSP), an atypical neurodegenerative disease that is underrecognized.[2] The insidious onset affects movement, gait, balance, speech, swallowing, vision, eye movement, mood, behavior, and cognition.[3] It is the most common parkinsonian disorder after Parkinson's disease (PD) that has an unusual constellation of supranuclear gaze palsy, progressive axial rigidity, pseudobulbar palsy, and mild dementia.[2-4] The cause of PSP is unknown, but what is recognized is the unfortunate response to medications and poor prognosis.[3]

As health care becomes increasingly valued in society, nurses will be expected to take more responsibility for health care delivery. It is obvious that there are gaps and priorities in the health care service that require an extension of nursing. Clinical nurse specialists (CNS) have a unique nursing role that can bridge the gaps in health care, especially for patients with PSP.

In PSP care, CNSs can demonstrate expertise by specializing in direct care that helps to improve patients' quality of life. To accomplish this, the CNS must educate patients, families, and other health care professionals on PSP management, symptom control and assist with care transitions.

Epidemiology

Progressive supranuclear palsy is a fatal disease.[2] In recent reports, the prevalence of PSP is 5 to 7 per 100,000 persons with an annual incidence density rate between 0.9 and 2.6 per 100,000 persons,[5] which equally escalate with age. The average age of onset ranges from 40 to 65 years of age[5]; life expectancy is variable, ranging from 5 to 7 years following the onset of symptom.[2-5] Conversely, patients' comorbidities can make life expectancy longer or shorter. What should be noted is that good interprofessional care embracing the expertise of a CNS may improve both the quality and length of life for those with PSP.

Nature of the Problem

Progressive supranuclear palsy is caused by the build-up of a protein called tau in certain areas of the brain and forms into clumps (neurofibrillary tangles).[3] The normal function of tau is to help support the microtubules. But when there is excess phosphate on the tau protein molecules, it causes the tau to misfold.[3] When it misfolds, it assumes a more rigid structure and clumps together. These clumps are toxic to the cell, which eventually die. Even before the cell dies, it releases misfolded, clumped tau protein into the fluid surrounding the cells. That tau is then taken up by neighboring healthy cells that undergo the same damaging chain reaction of tau misfolding, templating, and clumping.[3] In this way, the process of brain cell malfunction and death spreads slowly through the brain. As a result, the regions of the brain that are related to balance, movement, vision, and speech die, causing an early loss of balance and falls, cognitive problems, and gaze palsy.[2] The signs and symptoms of PSP are triggered by a progressive deterioration of midbrain cells, causing the initiation of impaired eye movement and balance.[6]

Clinical Characteristics

Many patients characteristically present to health care providers with disequilibrium, unsteadiness, and dizziness with unexplained falls.[7] To rule out other diagnoses, patients should be assessed for an inner ear disturbance. The classic symptom of supranuclear gaze is an abnormality of extraocular eye movements that is usually present[2,6–8];however, it may not be seen initially due to reasons why patients sought health care in the first place; falls. Neck and lower extremity muscle rigidity are frequently present.[6] Usually, the patient is diagnosed with atypical parkinsonian disorder, yet, as PSP progresses, the vision is affected; the patient generally experiences blurred or double vision.[9] The hallmark feature is paralysis of the nuclei causing the restriction of the patients up and downward gaze.[9,10] This inadequate supranuclear connection precludes the patient from moving his/her eyes voluntarily. Patients have what is known as "the doll's eye reflex," which is also known as the vestibular ocular reflex.[11] This reflex can be elicited by moving the patient's head passively while watching their gaze, which is fixated on an object. Unfortunately, the production of the vestibular ocular reflex is an indication of poor brainstem function.[11] Because the vertical eye movements are typically more altered than the horizontal movements, the impairment is assessed with the downward gaze. In later PSP stages, the gaze can be affected in all directions.

Because focusing the eyes properly is the main difficulty, reading becomes challenging because of the inability to automatically shift the eyes down from line to line.[2] Likewise, the patient may not be able to see food on a plate or an object in the path when walking. Later in the disease process, horizontal gaze paresis, eyelid apraxia, blepharospasms, and severely reduced blinking occurs.[11] Another common visual problem that families find frustrating is the inability of patients with PSP to maintain eye contact during conversation.[2,11] This gives the mistaken impression that the patient is senile, hostile, or uninterested.

As the disease progresses, the patient develops the classic appearance of sustained surprise, which is exhibited as either a startled facial expression or a stone face due to contracted facial muscles.[12] Speech becomes slurred in most patients with irregularity; at times, it may be spastic or ataxic speech.[6,8,10] Mental slowness occurs; sleep disturbances, angry outbursts, impaired judgment, apathy, and depression can create an erroneous impression of senility.[2,4–6] Further disease progression leads to feeding difficulties. Swallowing foods or thin liquids can become problematic because of throat muscle weakness or incoordination.[2,13] Patients tend to overload the mouth or to take big gulps of beverages due to a loss of inhibition or reckless impulsiveness, causing choking or aspiration.[13] Unfortunately, aspiration pneumonia is the most common cause of death in PSP.[2]

At the time of diagnosis, a supporting family member or care partner should be present, relevant written information should be provided, and a plan of care with the interprofessional team should be made. During disease progression, patients typically present with loss of balance and unexplained falls, impacting the activities of daily living. The patient may experience minor difficulties with complex fine motor tasks such as writing, tying shoelaces, and fastening buttons.[2] There may be some slowness of movement, and balance is often unsteady, resulting in backward falls.[6–9] They are also at an increase in postural reactions, which become progressively impaired with a tendency toward risky movement, such as motor recklessness, lurching gait, clumsiness leading to frequent falls, uncontrolled impulsivity and choking while continuing to ingest food.[2,8] This, with increasing muscle rigidity, may lead to immobility and very limited movement of the extremities. The focus of support should be on independence, prevention, and safety.

PROGRESSIVE SUPRANUCLEAR PALSY COMORBIDITIES

Patients who suffer from PSP also have numerous comorbidities consisting of neurological and musculoskeletal disorders such as gait and motility issues, speech impairment, and dysphagia with a secondary diagnosis of pneumonia; cardiovascular complications such as essential hypertension, and urological problems, including incontinence, urgency, and frequency.[13] Therefore, patients with PSP should be assessed for these comorbidities to circumvent these additional factors that may intensify the central nervous system's neurodegenerative burden. Concerning appropriate patient care, an accurate patient assessment is necessary.

Nursing Care

There may be times when patients with PSP are admitted to the intensive care unit (ICU). These patients have family members who are their primary care partners performing the activities of daily living; bathing, dressing, and feeding. Without full patient support, ambulation is impossible. Communication is usually with nods, thumbs up or down, and facial expressions that family members have learned to understand. Just because patients with PSP are trapped inside their failing bodies, they understand everything that is happening to and around them. Therefore, the aim of care should reflect life maintenance.

Nurses working in the ICU combine scientific knowledge with advanced technologies while humanizing individual care, thus contributing to improved patient outcomes and experiences. Since PSP is progressive, patients who spend time in the ICU, usually have a diagnosis of choking or aspiration. Therefore, nurses specializing in the ICU must be aware of what PSP is along with symptom management for proper care coordination.

Because ICU nurses are uniquely trained and use knowledge to assess changing conditions, interpret laboratory values, assess patients' hemodynamic status, titrate medications accordingly, and manage multiple devices, they optimize patient care. Once the PSP patient is hemodynamically stable, they are transferred to a lower level of care or home. ICU nurses organize and perform PSP patient transfers in the continuum of care to ensure minimal disruptions, yet it can be challenging. Although the care transition may be desirable, the journey from the ICU to lower-level care or home can be hazardous and frustrating for patients with PSP and family members.

Nurses working in the ICU can employ patient and family strategies to contribute to a safe, secure, collaborative, and successful care transition. For instance, ICU nurses can include activities to preserve patient safety and prevent adverse events during the transfer. These activities can focus on reducing intensive care (technology and medication administered), encouraging self-ability, customizing information, and arranging a pretransfer meeting to collaborate and communicate with all interprofessional team members, including patients and families. Likewise, ICU nurses can support patients' own self-care ability with sensitivity by strengthening, inspiring, and giving hope and courage to patients and families; their participation matters. It is important to note that encouragement is repeatedly needed, along with patient/family-specific customized information, including several notifications about the transition progress, times, and goals; this may decrease their apprehension. With communication, coordination, and collaboration between the three parties; nurses and patient/family, interprofessional team members and involved units, and patient/family and environment. By preparing the patient and family for care transition, the multifaceted process ensures the necessary continuity of care.[14]

Transition of Care

Since the transition of care is multifaceted, it can cause concern for patients with PSP and their families. As reported in research, patients that undergo care transition are at an increased risk of ICU-acquired skeletal muscle mass wasting,[15] post ICU mind, body and emotional symptoms,[15] and morbidity and mortality[15] along with frequently enduring poor communication and inconsistent care.[16] Patients with PSP and their families worry about the uncertainty in care, including who is accountable for their care and what is available regarding care resources. They may feel overwhelmed. However, the success of the care transition depends on the hospital's efforts and the health care team's coordination and support. Nurses serve as a primary and trusted source of information and support for patients and families during the transition of care. By virtue of their role and expertise, CNSs can support and guide patients with PSP and families and ICU nurses in successful care transition.

Clinical Nurse Specialist Considerations

Although patients with PSP suffer from balance instability, visual impairments, impulsivity, and swallowing issues, utilizing CNSs in the ICU and for care transitions would be beneficial, and by joining the interprofessional team, they can assess and recommend specialized care for these patients to receive. By doing so, the CNS contributes to patient outcomes by identifying problems and providing high-level practice through decision support and team building for dealing with difficult problems and patients in complex situations.[16] They can exert their expertise through three spheres of impact; patient/family, nurse/ health care professionals, and the health care organization. They also apply the seven core competencies to nursing-based care; direct care, consultation, system leadership, collaboration, coaching, research, and ethical decision-making.[17] Because of their contribution to patient care, it raises the stature of nursing care by assisting with the development of expertise in nursing care in specific specialized areas, such as patients with PSP admitted to the ICU. Likewise, CNSs support stakeholders (ie, patients with PSP and all ICU health care providers) in addressing patients with PSP, their clinical problems, and managing their care and treatment with research-based practice guidelines, leading to quality patient outcomes. Additionally, CNSs who understand patients with PSP can create evidence-based care pathways, use culturally sensitive communication, and implement care changes and improvements in nursing and interprofessional staff practices, striving for a successful care transition.

Patient/family sphere of impact

CNSs practicing in the sphere of patient/family recognize that the fundamental success of care transition is the universal need for compassionate communication and empathy. This is characterized by both the patient's and family members' experience of how care was delivered. Because this element is based on the care transition experience, it is tightly linked to the overarching goal of feeling cared for and cared about. Therefore, CNSs understand that when patients with PSP and care partners report poor care experiences, they are saying that health care teams lack empathy and compassion. When patients and family members feel ignored or disregarded in the process of making decisions regarding care transitions, they feel misaligned, and decisions remain unclear. This failure to work collaboratively with patients and family members impedes inclusivity and lacks attentiveness, support, and compassion.[14,15] CNSs can develop expertise in compassionate communication. Once accomplished, they should plan for disseminating this information and have all health care staff practice such soft skills.

CNSs recognize that there is a requirement to anticipate PSP patients' transitional care needs, medical equipment, medications, education, and appropriate transportation. This is a fiduciary responsibility; there is a duty to ensure that the patient avoids complications or adverse events, as well as preventable returns to the ICU/ health care organization. When CNSs involve the patient/family member collaboratively with the discharge planning, it makes the participants feel a sense of support and caring, ensuring that they are prepared for the care transition and are capable of carrying out the care plan. If patients and family members are not involved, they feel disregarded and perceive a feeling of apprehension and weariness that their specific plans of care were not addressed.[18] This is concerning since patients with PSP have numerous complex needs, and the specific care provisions must be met to obtain quality of life. Intensive Care Unit CNSs working with patients with PSP and families can provide specialized care for such needs that are tailored, easily understandable, and execute training on specific clinical skills prior to the transition. If this does not happen, patients and family members will struggle to adhere to plans, causing transitional anxiety, making the experience overwhelming and stressful, along with the feeling of being deserted by the health care team. For example, CNSs can prepare patients and family members on fall safety preventative measures and aspiration pneumonia precautions. Training family members on how to avoid harm to their loved ones while eating and ambulating can ensure a successful care transition. When patients and family members are fully prepared to handle potential complications, they have less emotional distress and feel prepared for the care needed during the transition.

Nurse/ health care provider sphere of impact

For patients with PSP and families, lack of health care provider knowledge is a priority concern.[18] This is distressing, especially in a crisis when patients with PSP and families seek care within the ICU environment. Unfortunately, the ICU climate usually has strict visiting policies, insisting that families cannot stay at the bedside. This antiquated approach to care allows the patient to be left alone, suffering in solitude around interprofessional teams who lack PSP knowledge. Since health care providers lack PSP knowledge, another family concern is the discovery that they must become competent in educating health care providers about PSP. However, when the family cannot be at the bedside of their loved one, the challenge of educating health care providers about the need for patience and compassion to care for such patients is a gap in responsibility. Because ICU care is a challenging environment with numerous illnesses, improving health care PSP knowledge will translate into more competent, timely, and supportive care for such patients.

To accomplish this, the Clinical Nurse Specialist can practice in the nurse/ health care provider sphere. CNSs can assist with optimal approaches to interprofessional team education, thus making significant contributions to PSP patient care. With educational interventions geared toward patients with PSP and families, CNSs should embrace the need to guide and support ICU nurses and health care providers with coaching, thus cultivating confidence in caring for such patient and family-specific complex needs.

To welcome a culture of engagement where patients and families are involved in all aspects of care, CNSs can engage at the personal, organizational, and macro level to guide policy change. This supports a physical environment that is conducive to patient-centeredness care. With this paradigm shift, CNSs ought to plan, deliver, manage, and improve patient and family partnerships in care by effectively communicating and actively listening, resulting in the enormous potential for sustained quality health care outcomes.

Likewise, if ICU nurses/ health care providers glean valuable insight into the impor- tance of effective communication and active listening skills from the CNS, they can implement these soft skills with complex patients with PSP ' and their transitional care. One avenue is to sit down and talk (and listen) with the patient/family throughout the ICU stay and about the transition; this creates a feeling of presence and demon- strates patience, compassion, and understanding. Then patients and families feel a commitment from the ICU nurse, making the challenging transition of care attentive, supportive, reliable, and with benevolence.

When health care is delivered in the absence of empathy, it is experienced as trans- actional. The typical consequences of dispassionate care precipitates and generates patient and family distress. It may also further deteriorate the patient's PSP condition, leading to care plan nonadherence and animosity toward the health care system. For these complex patients with PSP and family members, treatment by health care teams, when delivering care transition, must be given with expertise and proper specialized care education with sensitivity.

Health Care Systems Sphere of Impact

CNSs practicing in the health care system sphere recognize that patients with PSP and families desire unambiguous accountability from the health care system through the point of care transitions. This outcome is explained as understanding who on the health care team (ie, nurses, physicians, and so forth.) is accountable for managing and guiding the plan of care and who is the point of contact for questions or advice during the care transition. Distinctly, this clear channel of responsibility and access to care can provide the patient and family members the needed reassurance, thus cultivating trust. It should be noted that a lack of accountability is underscored when patients and families have unreliable mechanisms to access health care pro- viders for advice or have questions that require answers following discharge. This leads to uncertainty, precipitated by ambiguous information about who is the resource person when concerns arise, resulting in feelings of abandonment during or after the care transition, thus, inducing anxiety, angst, and mistrust.[19] CNSs can effectively communicate the plan of care for transition, providing actionable information along with clear and concise discharge instructions, including a point of contact for when concerns arise. This continuity in care cultivates a sense of being when patients are known as a person; this creates greater confidence, engagement, and trust in the health care system.

Since CNSs influence patient care at every level of inpatient hospital stays, they are promoters of synthesized research and its application to practice; they role model care and provide compassionate consultation to complex patients requiring special- ized care. Because CNSs practice exclusively in specific areas of the hospital setting, Intensive Care Unit CNSs can diagnose, care for, treat, and manage complex patients with PSP. To do so, they promote all 3 spheres of impact by managing PSP specialty patients, educating and supporting health care providers, and facilitating changes in care transitions within the organization.

The CNS can also serve as a bridge during the transition of care in the hospital, ensuring that communication is effective, care is consistent, and patient resources are readily available. The CNS can also partner with the patient and the family to plan for discharge care transition, including ongoing assessment and recommenda- tions. This is where the role of the CNS can have an impact; the utilization of their expertise is essential in linking and optimizing complex care to other health care pro- viders who may not have cared for patients with PSP before. When CNSs enhance the education of health care providers and place the patient in the appropriate level of care, it speaks to the principle of beneficence. Collaboration with a consultative ICU CNS nursing approach develops, models, and builds the competency of the bedside nurse and allows for patients with PSP ' specific needs without compromise.

SUMMARY

The journey of PSP is complex, difficult, and challenging, without any hope of a cure. However, many aspects of care are manageable. Effective management starts with achieving an early, accurate diagnosis. Without an accurate diagnosis, there are delays in patient care, resulting in delayed quality of care. The diagnosis is not difficult; does the patient have a tendency to fall?, do they walk with their head up and ridged? do their eyes appear as staring' with an odd, fixed smile?, do they have a distorted, slow, and effortful speech? There can be personality changes; are they impulsive?; this results from cognitive impairments in PSP.

Unfortunately, PSP robs individuals of many abilities and aspirations, but health care providers often unwittingly remove the patient's autonomy. Patient-centered treatment and care transition is more satisfying and more likely to succeed. A great source of frustration that undermines the confidence of patients and family members is not being a part of the collaborative team.

CNSs can be instrumental in the care of the PSP patient through their knowledge of the disease; they can communicate with other health care providers, the patient, and the family, supporting the care needed during this painful journey and the transition of care experience. If the health care experience is positive for patients with PSP and families, the transition of care is continuous and consistent with compassionate care and accountability. The benefits of effective communication, shared decision-making, continuity of care, and the anticipation of patients' and family needs are integral components of care transition, leading to better adherence. Negative PSP care transition experiences involve care perceived as transactional, leaving patients and families feeling fearful and abandoned, creating mistrust, anxiety, and confusion.

For patients with PSP, it should be noted that there is a serious gap that exists between the services needed and the services provided during these transitions. CNSs embracing the 3 spheres of impact can help bridge the gap by assisting the health care organization, patient, and families to better prepare for care transition and design accessible channels for ongoing support in order to ensure the journey from the ICU to other units and/or home is safe and supports each person's quality of life. It is the hope that clear accountability, care continuity, and caring attitudes are practiced and demonstrated as these are the essential health care needs of patients with PSP and family members as they navigate care transitions.

CLINICS CARE POINTS

- Progressive Supranuclear Palsy (PSP) is fatal and requires complex care management.

- Clinical Nurse Specialists (CNS) can apply the 3 spheres of impact by addressing health care concerns for patients with PSP and assist with care transition, recognizing specialty needs.

- By navigating care and addressing transition gaps for patients with PSP, CNSs can assist patients and families with the quality of life and life maintenance with supportive resources.

- Intensive Care Unit nurses can employ patient and family strategies to contribute to a safe, secure, collaborative, and successful care transition.

REFERENCES

1. Adams J, Zimmermann D. Setting a strategy for advancing nursing's influence. Journal for Nurses in Professional Development 2022;38(5):308–10.
2. Golbe LI. A clinician's guide to progressive supranuclear palsy. New Brunswick, NJ: Rutgers University Press; 2018.
3. Coughlin DG, Irene L. Progressive supranuclear palsy: advances in diagnosis and management. Park Relat Disord 2020;73:105–16.
4. Wen Y., Zhou Y., Jiao B., et al., Genetics of progressive supranuclear palsy: a review, *J Parkinsons Dis*, 11, 2021, 93–105.
5. Barer Y, Chodick G, Cohen R, et al. Epidemiology of Progressive Supranuclear Palsy: real world data from the second largest health plan in Israel. Brain Sci 2022;12:1126.
6. Giagkou N, Günter U. Höglinger, and maria stamelou. "Progressive supranuclear palsy". Int Rev Neurobiol 2019;149:49–86.
7. Smith MD, Ben-Shlomo Y, Henderson E. How often are patients with Progressive Supranuclear Palsy really falling? J Neurol 2019;266:2073–4.
8. Morgan JC, Ye X, Mellor JA, et al. Disease course and treatment patterns in Progressive Supranuclear Palsy: a real-world study. J Neurol Sci 2021;421:117293.
9. Debnath M., Dey S., Sreenivas N., et al., Genetic and epigenetic constructs of progressive supranuclear palsy, *Ann Neurosci*, 29 (2–3), 2022, 177–188.
10. Ticku H, Fotedar N, Juncos J, et al. Pseudonystagmus in progressive supranuclear palsy. J Neurol Sci 2022;434:120157.
11. Fabbrini G, Fabbrini A, Suppa A. Progressive Supranuclear Palsy, multiple system atrophy and corticobasal degeneration. Handb Clin Neurol 2019;165: 155–77.
12. Enver N., Borders J.C., Curtis J., et al., The role of vocal fold bowing on cough and swallowing dysfunction in Progressive Supranuclear Palsy, *Laryngoscope*, 131 (6), 2021, 1217–1222.
13. Zella M.A.S., Bartig D., Herrmann L., et al., Hospitalization rates and comorbidities in patients with progressive supranuclear palsy in Germany from 2010 to 2017, *J Clin Med*, 9 (8), 2020, 2454.
14. Häggström M, Bäckström B. Organizing safe transitions from intensive care. Nursing and Research Practice 2014;2014:175314.
15. Frampton SB, Guastello S, Hoy L, et al. Harnessing evidence and experience to change culture: a guiding framework for patient and family engaged care. NAM perspectives. Washington, DC: Discussion Paper, National Academy of Medicine; 2017. https://doi.org/10.31478/201701f.
16. Black BP. Professional nursing: concepts & challenges. 9th edition. St. Louis, MO: Elsevier; 2020.
17. Joseph J. Factors influencing the implementation of nurse specialist in health care management of a tertiary level hospital. Nurs J India 2020;111(5):225–30.
18. Moore T, Guttman M. Challenges faced by patients with progressive supranuclear palsy and their families. Movement Disorders Clinical Practice 2014;1(3): 188–93.
19. Respondek G, Breslow D, Amirghiasvand C, et al. The lived experiences of people with progressive supranuclear palsy and their caregivers. Neurol Ther 2023; 12(1):229–47.

The Sensitive Care of the Elder Orphan in Critical Care Environments

Rebekah LaDuke, MSN-NE, APRN, AG-ACCNS, CCRN[a],
Jennifer Rotter, MSN, APRN, AGCNS-BC, CCRN-K[b],*

KEYWORDS

- Medical durable power of attorney • Critical care • Elderly • Elder orphan • ICU

KEY POINTS

- Elder orphans are a growing vulnerable population who pose increased concerns to delivery of care at all levels and types.
- Elder orphans need to be identified out in the community before hospitalization or identfied upon admission to the hospital.
- Elder orphans require consults to case management and social work immediately to assist in finding legal next of kin or the legal process to obtain guardianship.
- Elder orphans require health-care insitutions to work with the community to establish plans and resources.

INTRODUCTION

The neurotrauma intensive care unit (NTICU) nurse comforts Sherrie, who has been Henrietta's home caregiver for the last 2 years. Henrietta has suffered from a severe ischemic stroke and subsequent aspiration pneumonitis. Sherrie is grieving because Henrietta's niece who lives nearly 3218.7 km away and who has only met her a few times throughout her life, had to make the long-distance decision over the phone to withdrawal life support. Sherrie reports feeling guilty that she was not with Henrietta when she had the stroke but instead found her laying on the bathroom floor with an unknown down time. Henrietta passes away quickly and peacefully after extubation but Sherrie and the critical care nursing staff are still saddened by the fact that a very distant, nonengaged, legal next of kin was the individual who had to make end of life and code status decisions for Henrietta.

---

[a] E.W. Sparrow Hospital, 1215 East Michigan Avenue, Lansing, MI 48912, USA; [b] Trinity Health Ann Arbor, Reichert Health Building, 5333 McAuley Drive, Suite 6003, Ypsilanti, MI 48197, USA
* Corresponding author.
E-mail address: Jenny.Rotter@trinity-health.org

Crit Care Nurs Clin N Am 35 (2023) 403–411
https://doi.org/10.1016/j.cnc.2023.05.005
0899-5885/23/© 2023 Elsevier Inc. All rights reserved.
ccnursing.theclinics.com

Sherrie came into Henrietta's life in the winter of 2021. It was January when Henrietta and her husband of 55 years, Bill, contracted coronavirus disease 2019 (COVID-19). Henrietta had moderate illness, required hospitalization but recovered and was discharged home. Bill unfortunately developed severe illness, was intubated, and eventually passed away. Before this, Henrietta and Bill were a relatively healthy married geriatric couple. They lived alone and supported each other with completing their activities of daily living (ADLs). Once home, Henrietta quickly realized that with Bill now gone and with the lingering fatigue, weakness, and shortness of breath she was experiencing after an acute hospitalization from COVID-19, she needed some day-to-day help.

This is when Sherrie came into the picture because Henrietta was suddenly and unexpectedly an elder orphan. She and Bill had one son who unfortunately had died in his 20s from a motor vehicle accident, thus leaving them with no immediate close relatives to act as a support system, caregiver, next of kin, let alone a durable power of attorney. Henrietta's distant family members had all relocated to the west coast decades ago. After the COVID-19 pandemic started, her connection with them had significantly dwindled due to everyone's decreased ability and/or willingness to travel. Henrietta and Sherrie had discussed on and off about designating someone to become Henrietta's medical durable power of attorney (MDPOA) but it ended up becoming incomplete because Henrietta just could not decide who would be the best choice. She always assumed Bill would be present for these types of challenging decisions.

BACKGROUND

More than 30 years ago, the discussion of orphaned elders emerged but was only utilized to describe individuals living out in the community who had cognitive impairments and difficult advocacy concerns.[1] Then throughout the decades, the term elder orphan emerged and started to evolve as more and more seniors were determined to be eligible under an "orphan" category. This continued until 2016, when Carney and colleagues[2] used the term elder orphan and gave it the formal definition of "aged, community-dwelling individuals who are socially and/or physically isolated, without an available known family member or designated surrogate or caregiver" (p.1). Although this definition is considered by most to be the gold standard, some criteria for elder orphan designation can vary. Generally, characteristics of this population consist of individuals who are aged older than 65 years and living independently out in the community without family or friends who can be consistently relied on for assistance when that need should arise.[3] Some groups have started to decrease the age criteria to as low as 55 years because individuals within this age range may have increased health-care support needs as well.[4]

Along with some varying diagnostics, terminology for this population can also vacillate. Unbefriended older adults, solo agers, kinless seniors, kinless older adults, isolated vulnerable adults, and adults without advocates, are all titles that can become intertwined and jumbled as synonyms for elder orphan.[1,5,6] However, what each of these means can differ between users because oftentimes there are slight nuances in definition. For example, an unbefriended older adult is referring to anyone who is unable to make their own medical decisions, advance directives, and who have no legal surrogate; however, it does not speak to their living arrangements or level of isolation.[1,6,7] There does seem within the literature a desire to focus on either an elderly patient's reported isolation or their lack of a legal surrogate, when in actuality these concerns commonly exist simultaneously. Thus, the vernacular of "elder orphan"

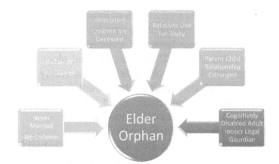

Fig. 1. Variable paths toward elder orphan criteria noted in literature.[1,2,5]

seems to address many more attributes than some of the other terms but being sensitive to the ongoing conversation that continues to happen around finding the most beneficial and compassionate term to describe the members of this vulnerable population is essential.

Titles aside, becoming an elder orphan is not usually intentional. The path to this designation can also vary as much as the final destination's title (**Fig. 1**).[1,2,5] As most individuals age, their parents pass away first. This leaves a person with their spouse and/or children to help them with complex health-care needs or other challenging ADLs in the later years of life. However, what happens when someone never marries and therefore does not have anyone legally attached to them for advocacy needs should he/she/they lose that capacity? There is a growing population of individuals who are choosing not to marry or have a civil union, not realizing that there are legal rights given to an individual when they become a lawfully recognized spouse. What if someone becomes a widow(er) and either never had children or their offspring have passed on before them, such as with Henrietta in the introductory story? Another path that is increasing in frequency is individuals who have immediate or distant family members but these relatives now live far away, possibly even in another country. Emotional support may be available from these individuals but relying on them for physical help cannot be expected.

Finally, there are some paths to elder orphan status that are not always considered. One being, someone who has children or other family members; however, because of substance abuse issues, criminal history, behavioral/mental health concerns, or due to a combination of these, the relationships have become estranged. This estrangement could be because the elder orphan suffers from social, behavioral, or legal problems or that they have distanced themselves because their family members were not considered "safe and healthy" to interact with. Another commonly forgotten path is an aging individual who has a cognitive disability who has lost their legal guardian, who is commonly a parent or sibling. An example could be an individual who has a significant cognitive delay since overcoming severe meningitis as a small child but who lives out in the community with the help of his/her/their sister who acts as their legal guardian. Yet should this legal guardian no longer be available for support or decision-making, the cognitively disabled adult can be suddenly orphaned.[5]

Prevalence/Incidence

The 2020 United States Census[8] shows that almost 17% of the population is aged older than 65 years. Of that group, more than 14 million individuals are being reported as living alone. Unfortunately, elder orphan data are not calculated but, in 2020,

Roofeh and colleagues[9] estimated that 2.62% of individuals aged older than 65 years could be considered an elder orphan by using data from the National Health and Aging Trends Survey. Utilizing this predetermined estimate and applying it to the 2020 census data would give the United States a potential elder orphan population of more than 360,000 persons. This would indicate how many people already meet orphaned status. Roofeh and colleagues[9] then went further to report the risk of becoming an elder orphan being estimated at 21.29%, which would leave another 2.9 million seniors at risk of becoming orphaned according to the US Census data. However, these estimates are most likely a gross underestimate because all the statistical figures were compiled before the COVID-19 pandemic had full effects. With the geriatric population seeing the majority of death within this country from a day-to-day basis during the pandemic, the world health crisis can then be considered an unexpected accelerant to the elder orphan population.

March 2023 marks the 3-year anniversary of the COVID-19 pandemic starting in the United States of America and the Centers for Disease Control and Prevention's[10] COVID-19 data tracker reported the United States as having 103,672,529 total contracted cases along with a staggering 1,119,762 deaths. More than 75% of these reported deaths fall within the population of individuals who are aged 65 years and older.[10] Therefore, it is reasonable to assume that an increase in elder orphans is quite possible. Additionally, the next age group of 50 to 64-year-olds made up another 17.6% of reported COVID-19 deaths.[10] This figure is significant because this age group will be trending to over the age of 65 in the next 15 years, thus making them again eligible for elder orphan status should they not have children, family members, or friends who are local and engaged within their life or, at the very least, have a designated caregiver or MDPOA established. With COVID-19 infections sometimes killing multiple individuals within the same family lineage and across generations, it is not unreasonable to think that even younger individuals may already be orphaned adults with no eligible next of kin.

So prevalent and growing is this subpopulation that support groups exist. One such digital support is the "Elder Orphan" Facebook page, which currently reports more than 10,000 group members. It has been in existence since 2016 for anyone aged older than 55 years who, "Live without the help of a spouse, partners, and children. If you feel you're aging alone with little support, you belong."[4] This highlights that not only are health-care institutions and providers recognizing this group but at the individual level, people are self-identifying as an orphaned elder and seeking support.

Clinical Relevance

Why should we worry? The Society of Critical Care Medicine[11] states more than 5 million patients are admitted to intensive care units annually across the United States with most of these patients being adults. Given the statistics discussed earlier, the population of elder orphans who will require intervention for a critical illness are only expanding. Although geriatric critical care patients are notoriously challenging to care for due to their complexity, adding in the obstacle of determining who will make life-altering decisions for them because they are either permanently or temporarily incapacitated only intensifies the challenges.

Medical Concerns

Lack of kin, caregivers, or predetermined MDPOAs leave health-care providers and health-care institutions in precarious positions that are troublesome. It can cause.

- Delays in care while waiting for next of kin or guardianship to be determined

Table 1
Elder orphan medical concern examples

Example 1: A 75-year-old woman comes in unresponsive. The neighbor called EMS when she heard the dog barking nonstop but reports not being close with the patient. Critical care team suspects urosepsis with acute renal failure. There is no chart of this patient, no medical history and no family or known next of kin. Patient is not responding well to sepsis treatments but the health-care team may not know that the patient takes lithium, and an admitting diagnosis of lithium toxicity should also be considered	*Example 2*: A 72-year-old man comes in with altered mental status when a senior meal delivery person called 911 for conditions of the residence. Patient is dehydrated, malnourished, and has hyponatremia. With rehydration and nutrition, the interdisciplinary team expects mentation to improve but it is not. Head CT was negative. With no history and no kin, the hospital is left doing extensive testing to find a possible cause for altered level of consciousness. Is it reversible like delirium or more progressive like dementia?

- Incomplete medical, surgical, social, and family histories
- Unknown medication/prescription lists
- Possibly missed known allergens
- Consents being signed by providers during emergency situations
- Increased length of stays in intensive care units (ICU) and overall hospitalization

The above obstacles in caring for elder orphans can have devastating consequences (**Table 1**). The lack of a prescribed and over-the-counter medication list and missing medical or surgical history can potentially leave the patient misdiagnosed and improperly treated. Additionally, although the above list and examples are most likely a very generalized summary of some of the medical challenges that develop when elder orphans are within critical care environments, it is frequently the ethical dilemmas that plague the health-care professionals the most.

Ethical Concerns

When a critically ill individual does not have adequate representation to advocate for them or their health-care wishes, some of the voiced concerns that intensive care professionals discuss include the following.

- Are we following the patient's wishes?

Table 2
Elder orphan ethical concern examples

Example 1: A 66-year-old man is admitted to the ICU for hypothermia and diabetes ketoacidosis after being found wondering around outside without proper attire in winter. History shows patient suffered from a traumatic brain injury more than 20 years ago. Lives with his 80-year-old mother who is his legal guardian but she was in the hospital last week and passed away from complications of influenza. No one can find who has been caring for this patient since his mother's death or what will happen to him once he is cleared to be discharged	*Example 2*: An 88-year-old woman comes in after cardiac arrest. She collapsed while at church. Members of the congregation told EMS her husband passed away 2 months ago and their 2 children both passed away from cancer a long time ago. No one at the church could speak to her code status or end-of-life care wishes. Patient was treated as full code and pulse was regained. Her myocardial infarction was treated but patient has an anoxic brain injury. Case management is struggling to find kin. Legal guardianship is next but could take months to obtain

- Are we prolonging their suffering?
- Are these long-distance relatives that we found the right people to make these important end-of-life decisions?
- Assigned legal guardians do not know this person any better than we do, are they equipped to make health-care decisions?
- Where will this individual go when they get discharged? They cannot go home.
- I wonder if they had any pets at home that they were responsible for?
- This care is futile but do the policies support us in withdrawing care without next of kin or MDPOA support?

These moral decisions then weigh heavily on the interprofessional team and can stay with members of the team long after their interaction with the patient has stopped (**Table 2**).

Whether medical or ethical, decision-making occurs for elder orphan without their participation and without the help of someone who is close to them, leaving the health-care personnel carrying the burdens. This is relevant both for the patient who is having strangers make life-altering choices for them and for the health-care professionals who must live with the decisions that they made for the patient. Interventions are thus required to help elevate these problems.

DISCUSSION

With the elder orphan population growing in this country both naturally and exponentially from the COVID-19 pandemic, primary health-care providers and geriatric health-care clinics must start identifying patients who fit elder orphan criteria early on. Addressing elder orphan concerns out in the community before acute illnesses and exacerbations of chronic illnesses develop will be essential for a smoother transition of care. However, until this process is seamless, health-care institutions must also start recognizing these patients on hospitalization admission. Admission assessment identification would allow for more immediate case management and social work consults to be placed. Early involvement of these special care services causes pivotal steps such as prompt determination of next of kin, identifying additional resources, and/or timely initiation of the legal guardianship process to be initiated.

Additionally, the interdisciplinary teams within acute care spaces, especially critical care environments, must start talking about this population during daily rounds. Utilizing proper terminology when discussing an elder orphan patient's plan of care will help ensure that the best decisions are made in determining next steps for the individual while waiting for clarification on who is best able to make decisions for the solo ager.[2–5] Understanding the obstacles an elder orphan is going to encounter because of lack of support may alter whether aggressive versus more conservative methods of treatment are chosen. Timelines of care may also be altered if waiting for estranged relatives to arrive from long-distance travel or while waiting for code status changes once a legal guardian is assigned.

Health-care institutions however will not be able to tackle this problem alone. Working with local, state, and federal agencies to develop legislation that offers aid and protection to this vulnerable group is vital. Moreover, partnering with other local leaders and organizations to create support programs and community awareness will also be essential to ensure these individuals are not forgotten. Speaking at churches and senior centers about this topic may help current elder orphans or friends and neighbors of elder orphans understand the next steps that can be taken to protect an orphaned elder before he/she/they find themselves critically ill and not able to advocate for themselves.

Along with community involvement, health care needs to conduct ongoing research on how to best identify orphaned elders along with finding viable, personable, safe, and cost-effective interventions to help combat this growing health-care concern. Carney and colleagues[2] published *Questions to Screen for Risk for Elder Orphan Status*, yet research verifying the reliability and validity of this screening tool could not be located. Additionally, Carney and colleagues[2] published the *Ten-Step Guide to Caring for an Elder Orphan* and again discussion on how to build this questionnaire with recommendations into electronic medical records or health-care providers' workflows are not occurring regularly.

Long-term outcomes for solo agers has only begun to scratch the surface with most research focusing on isolated seniors having poor long-term health outcomes and increased mortality, with the causes being linked to both physical and social isolation and emotional loneliness.[12–15] Research showcasing whether elder orphans have an increased risk of chronic illness diagnoses or even acute emergency illnesses is missing. Are there differences between recovering from an acute illness versus an exacerbation for this group? Do solo agers have increased speed in which the progression of a chronic illness occurs or is it completely dependent on the individual? Research into these questions and their results could help propel the need for identifying individuals within this population sooner and thus attempt to mitigate poor outcomes.

Roofeh and colleagues[3] looked at the risk of elder orphans needing assisted living residence placement after an acute care hospitalization. The research has shown positive correlations between elder orphan criteria and an increased need for facility residence placement. This is a wonderful start but further research correlating this increased need of residential placement after hospitalization in a postpandemic environment is now warranted. After the COVID-19 pandemic, there have been fewer residential facility beds available to meet the demand for the growing elder orphan population on top of those seniors who may have support but family are still unable to assist due to complexity of the loved one's illness(es). This problem then extends hospital lengths of stay, which causes delays in transfers of care within the hospital thus lengthening stays in ICUs and emergency rooms across the nation. The American Hospital Association[16] published a brief in December of 2022 trying to quantify the bed capacity issue and reported that hospitals' average length of stay has increased by 19.2% since 2019 and that when extrapolating data for just those individuals who are waiting for long-term care bed options the increase is almost 24% since 2019.

Finally, research that looks at both acute care and community offerings and how to bridge support to elder orphans across health-care environments must happen. People want to age in their own personal living arrangements for as long as possible, so how do communities and health care work together to make sure this can happen safely for individuals with less physical or financial support? What programs exist, how are they funded, and most importantly are they meeting the needs of the elder orphans they serve?

SUMMARY

All patients within critical care units and environments are vulnerable. They are often either biologically unable to communicate their wishes and needs to their caregivers or rather their caregivers must temporarily strip them from these abilities pharmaceutically and/or mechanically while treating their acute critical illness. This inability to communicate is why interdisciplinary intensive care teams across the country heavily rely on spouses, children, siblings, parents, other next of kin, or other designated MDPOAs to advocate for those who cannot advocate for themselves. Unfortunately, there is a growing population of elder orphans who lack this support system when they need it the most. The statistics before COVID-19 were staggering for the inevitable growth of this vulnerable group but now the potential that elder orphans will be seen even more within critical care units after the pandemic is higher. Being cognizant to the complexities and challenges that this brings into the intensive care environment is essential so that sensitive care can be delivered even in the absence of a traditional familial support system. Conversations must begin on how we assess, identify, treat, and provide long-term services to those who no longer have it naturally.

CLINICS CARE POINTS

- Elder orphans are a growing vulnerable population
- Elder orphans within critical care environment pose increased concerns to delivery of care at all levels and types
- Elder orphans need to be identified out in the community before hospitalization
- Elder orphans not identified before hospitalization must be identified on admission
- Elder orphans require consults to case management and social work immediately to start the process of finding legal next of kin or the legal process to obtain guardianship
- Elder orphans require health-care institutions to work with the community to establish plans and resources

DECLARATION OF CONFLICTING INTERESTS AND FUNDING

The author(s) declare no potential commercial or financial conflicts of interest exist with respect to the authorship and/or publication of this article. Neither author received funding for this study.

REFERENCES

1. Kervin LM, Chamberlain SA, Wister AV, et al. (Older) Adults without advocates: support for alternative terminology to "elder orphan" in research and clinical contexts. J Am Geriatr Soc 2022;70(11):3329–33.
2. Carney MT, Fugiwara J, Emmert BE, et al. Elder orphans hiding in plain sight: a growing vulnerable population. Current Gerontology and Geriatrics Research 2016;4723250.
3. Roofeh R, Clouston SAP, Smith DM. Completing risk analysis of time to communal residence for elder orphans. J Appl Gerontol 2022;41(9):2105–12.
4. Francis J. Elder orphans on Facebook: implications for mattering and social isolation. Comput Hum Behav 2022;127:107023.
5. Montayer J, Thaggard S, Carney M. Views on the use of the term 'elder orphans': a qualitative study. Health Soc Care Community 2019;28:341–6.
6. Thaggard S, Montayre J. Elder orphans' experiences of advance planning and informal support network. SAGE Open; 2019. p. 1–6. https://doi.org/10.1177/2158244019865371.
7. Farrell TW, Wildera E, Rosenberg L, et al. AGS position statement: making medical treatment decisions for unbefriended older adults. J Am Geriatric Soc 2017;65(1):14.
8. United States Census Bureau (2023). Data profiles. Retrieved March 2023 from: Available at: https://www.census.gov/programs-surveys/decennial-census/decade/2020/2020-census-main.html.

9. Roofeh R, Clouston SAP, Smith DM. Estimated prevalence of elder orphans using national health and aging trends study. J Aging Health 2020;32(10):1443–9. https://journals.sagepub.com/doi/10.1177/0898264320932382.
10. Centers for disease Control and Prevention (CDC). COVID Data Tracker. Retrieved March 2023 from: Available at: https://covid.cdc.gov/covid-data-tracker/#datatracker-home.
11. Society of Critical Care Medicine SCCM. Critical care statistics. Retrieved March 2023 from: Available at: https://www.sccm.org/Communications/Critical-Care-Statistics.
12. Chan E, Procter-Gray E, Churchill L, et al. Elder orphans hiding in plain sight: a growing vulnerable population. Current Gerontology and Geriatrics Research 2016;2016:4723250.
13. Djundeva M, Dykstra PA, Fokkema T. Is living alone "aging alone"? Solitary living, network types, and well-being. Journals of Gerentology. Series B, Psychological Sciences 2019;74(8):1406–15.
14. Sakurai R, Yasunaga M, Nishi M, et al. Coexistence of social isolation and home-bound status increase the risk of all-cause mortality. Int Psychogeriatr 2019;31(5): 703–11.
15. Soones T, Federman A, Leff B, et al. Two-year mortality in homebound older adults: an analysis of the national health and aging trends study. J Am Geriatr Soc 2017;65(1):123–9.
16. American Hospital Association (AHA). Issue brief: Patients and providers faced with increasing delays in timely discharges. 2022; 1-2. Retrieved March 2023 from: Available at: https://www.aha.org/system/files/media/file/2022/12/Issue-Brief-Patients-and-Providers-Faced-with-Increasing-Delays-in-Timely-Discharges.pdf.

The Role and Initiatives Led by the Sepsis Coordinator to Improve Sepsis Bundle Compliance and Care Across the Continuum

Teresa Cranston, MSN, RN, CCRN-K[a],
Katharine Thompson, BA, MSN, RN-BC, AG-CNS[b],*,
Kathryn H. Bowles, PhD, RN[c]

KEYWORDS

- Severe sepsis • Septic shock • Sepsis core measures • CMS SEP-1 • CMS SEP-3
- Fluid resuscitation • Organ dysfunction • Sepsis criteria

KEY POINTS

- Dedicated sepsis coordinator to identify needs for new workflow processes to improve sepsis care across the continuum.
- Multidisciplinary team approach improves sepsis bundle compliance.
- Improving postacute transition of care reduces sepsis readmissions.

BACKGROUND

Sepsis is the body's acute systemic inflammatory response to an infection. It is a life-threatening clinical syndrome that can cause injury to the body's own tissues and organs.[1] Without early recognition and timely treatment, organ dysfunction caused by the body's dysregulated response to the infection can lead to death.[2] Sepsis is the leading cause of preventable death worldwide. The World Health Organization estimates sepsis affects 49 million people with 11 million deaths yearly.[3] In the United States, 1.7 million adults a year are diagnosed, with an estimated 350,000 hospitalized and home hospice deaths.[2]

More than 85% of sepsis cases are present on hospital admission.[1] The difficulty with sepsis recognition is that many illnesses present with the same signs and

[a] Penn Medicine Lancaster General Hospital, 555 North Duke Street, Lancaster, PA 17602, USA;
[b] Penn Medicine Lancaster General Hospital, 555 North Duke Street, Lancaster, PA 17602, USA;
[c] University of Pennsylvania, University of Pennsylvania School of Nursing, 418 Curie Boulevard, Claire M. Fagin Hall, Room 340, Philadelphia, PA 19104, USA
* Corresponding author.
E-mail address: Katharine.thompson@pennmedicine.upenn.edu

Crit Care Nurs Clin N Am 35 (2023) 413–424
https://doi.org/10.1016/j.cnc.2023.05.006
0899-5885/23/© 2023 Elsevier Inc. All rights reserved.
ccnursing.theclinics.com

symptoms. Clinical indicators can be elusive, especially in older adults and those individuals who are immunocompromised.[4] It is essential that clinicians practice routine sepsis screening to improve early recognition and rapid initiation of treatment with fluid resuscitation and antibiotics to improve patient outcomes. According to Sepsis Alliance, each hour of delayed antibiotic treatment is associated with a mortality increase of 4% to 9% in severe sepsis cases.[5]

In 2004, The Surviving Sepsis Campaign (SSC) published best practice guidelines for 3-hour and 6-hour bundle compliance to improve patient outcomes for severe sepsis and septic shock. In 2015, updated SSC bundles were adopted by The Centers for Medicare and Medicaid Services (CMS) as sepsis core measure (SEP-1) to help prevent the progression of sepsis to septic shock.[6,7] SEP-1 actions involves blood cultures, lactate levels, fluid resuscitation, antibiotics, and vasopressors to be ordered at 3-hour and 6-hour time intervals. CMS implementation of SEP-1 requires hospitals to measure SEP-1 compliance because hospital reimbursement/incentive payments are decided based on compliance to sepsis care. The core measures are evidence-based quality measurements mandated by CMS for standards of care and treatment processes to improve patient outcomes.[8]

The aim of this article is to describe how the value-added role of a sepsis coordinator created a sepsis program to improve SEP-1 compliance and transition of care for sepsis survivors. The coordinator's idea to use the continuous monitoring unit (CMU) for sepsis monitoring initiated a new nurse-driven workflow process to improve early recognition, treatment interventions, and postacute transition care resources. The sepsis coordinator's ability to advance collaboration with interprofessional teams has improved sepsis care across the continuum by decreasing mortality and reducing readmissions.

WHY A SEPSIS COORDINATOR?

The decision to create a sepsis coordinator role was based on the inability of various oversight committees to improve SEP-1 compliance and reduce readmissions. The lack of a centralized focus on sepsis care coordination and support for both providers and patients necessitated a sepsis coordinator to provide management and to develop new workflow processes to close gaps and provide follow through care for sepsis survivors. Sepsis is a very complicated and high-risk disease process, and it is not only important to capture early recognition but also imperative to follow these patients to their next level of care. Improving transitions is as important as early recognition and treatment.

The sepsis coordinator works in collaboration with all entities that touch the sepsis patient. When first building a sepsis program, it is necessary to not only look at organizational goals but also understand how and why current state processes are in place by starting with cases that originate in the emergency department. What does sepsis presentation look like? How do providers determine a patient is septic? How do abstraction rules determine the start time for core measure compliance?

IMPROVING SEPSIS CORE MEASURE COMPLIANCE
Abstraction

Understanding the CMS SEP-1 bundle compliance can be challenging, and the guidelines are strict and difficult to conquer. The SEP-1 bundle is a 3-hour and 6-hour set of rules that must be achieved within the set time frame. They seem straight forward but the difficulty is the start time or "time zero." Three components must be met within a 6-hour window: documentation of a suspected or verified infection, 2 or more systemic inflammatory response syndrome (SIRS) criteria, and one or more organ dysfunction criteria. Time zero is also activated if the provider documents severe sepsis or septic shock. The challenge is the varying determination of "time zero" by abstractors versus clinical workflows of clinicians, affecting whether the case may or may not meet sepsis compliance.[9]

At the time of the sepsis coordinator hire, SEP-1 compliance was at 45% with a goal rate of 55%. A significant point to highlight is the organization made the commitment to abstract every sepsis case for submission to CMS. Most organizations submit a sampling, which allows for a higher compliance rate to be achievable. The decision to submit every case was based on the need to ascertain why cases fell out so that opportunities for improvement could be tracked and monitored.[10] There by, it holds our organization to higher standards for our sepsis population. For improved alignment with CMS guidelines, the sepsis coordinator shadowed in-house abstractors and reviewed every abstraction case to better understand how start times were determined and reasons for delays in interventions.

Early Recognition

Rapid recognition of sepsis is essential for early treatment and improved outcomes. The difficulty with sepsis recognition is that many illnesses not only present with the same signs and symptoms of other underlying disease processes but also sepsis has significant variations among individuals with multiple comorbidities.[11,12] In older adults, sepsis can present with atypical syndrome-specific signs and symptoms requiring a higher awareness of a potentially underlying infection.[5] The complexities of sepsis response and recognition require biomarkers, diagnostic imaging, and clinical assessment. It is key that clinicians practice collaboration and communication when diagnosing and treating patients that may present with possible sepsis. Early detection, monitoring, and interventions are key to excellent care of the septic patient.[7] It takes carefully trained clinicians to dismiss the irrelevant and align the significant data.

The first step in the process was to help the frontline staff recognize signs and symptoms of sepsis. A sepsis best practice advisory (BPA) was created based on the SEP-1 definition, 2 SIRS criteria, and 1 organ dysfunction caused by an infection. A BPA is an electronic health record (EHR) alert that helps to identify possible infection; however, critical judgment is essential to determine between a chronic disease process and a true infection. For example, an international normalized ratio (INR) greater than 1.5 will trigger a BPA to fire, yet the provider needs to establish if elevation is due to sepsis, chronic disorder, or anticoagulation therapy.

Sepsis Recognition Tool

It was imperative that the frontline staff understood true organ dysfunction. To that end, the Penn Sepsis Alliance created and launched the Penn Medicine Sepsis Recognition Tool. The tool identified what the SIRS criteria and organ dysfunction criteria were with the clinical parameters. To roll out use of the tool, the sepsis coordinator led education sessions for providers and nursing staff. Educating nurses on early recognition of organ dysfunction was needed to facilitate the nurses' role in escalating communication for action by providers. In addition, a laminated badge buddy was created based on the Penn Medicine Sepsis Recognition Tool on one side and Required Actions per CMS SEP-1 on the other (**Fig. 1**). This badge assists the frontline staff in identifying true organ dysfunction as well as all required components of the SEP-1 core measures, including what is needed within the 3-hour and 6-hour bundle to meet compliance.

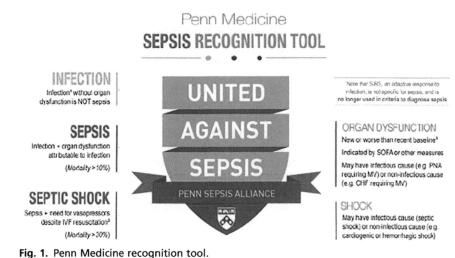

Fig. 1. Penn Medicine recognition tool.

Sepsis Order Set Modifications

Sepsis Order Sets were created and are reviewed biannually to stay up to date with CMS SEP-1 Core Measure guidelines based on the SSC recommendations:

- Blood cultures ×2 within 3 hours of sepsis recognition, before intravenous antibiotic administration
- Serum lactate level within 3 hours of sepsis recognition and repeat in 4 hour as needed if greater than 2.0 to capture the 6-hour deadline
- Broad spectrum intravenous antibiotics within 3 hours of sepsis recognition
- Crystalloid fluids of 30 mL/kg for body mass index (BMI) less than 30 or utilization of ideal body weight (IBW) for BMI greater than 30 for persistent hypotension and/or a lactate 4 or greater
- Vasopressors for persistent hypotension that is not fluid responsive
- Documentation of the Sepsis Reassessment within 6 hours of the recognition of septic shock

Early reviews into abstracted cases identified a proportionally higher fallout rate for the intravenous fluid (IVF) component. This was due to provider's clinical experience to prevent fluid overload for an already compromised patient.[13] In many cases, achieving the 30 mL/kg goal within 3 hours of a patient meeting criteria for septic shock would be challenging. The sepsis coordinator worked with the pharmacy team to create specialized orders to focus on BMI and IBW. If a patient had a BMI greater than 30, the orders would be based on the IBW providing a limit to IVF administration. Moreover, many of our septic patients had comorbid conditions that included heart or renal failure, which put them at higher risk for fluid overload. It was decided early on that the provider would document for the reason for limited IVF. It was still considered a missed resuscitation by CMS but it was recognized as reasonable judgment.

In 2021, CMS adopted the recommendation of the SSC, which allowed for IVF limits if there were documented concerns for fluid overload. This prompted further modifications to the order set to incorporate adjustment to the IVF options (**Fig. 2**). Again, our colleagues in pharmacy agreed to assist and created a stat pharmacy consult as well as a new order that would provide at least 15 mL/kg of IVF for the patient. The

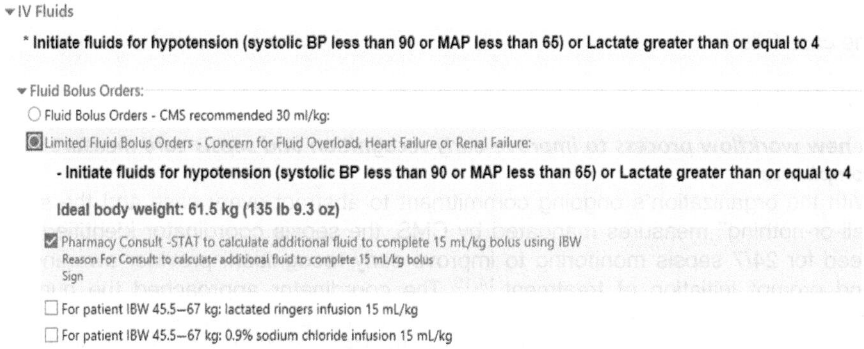

▼ IV Fluids

 * **Initiate fluids for hypotension (systolic BP less than 90 or MAP less than 65) or Lactate greater than or equal to 4**

 ▼ Fluid Bolus Orders:
  ○ Fluid Bolus Orders - CMS recommended 30 ml/kg:
  ◉ Limited Fluid Bolus Orders - Concern for Fluid Overload, Heart Failure or Renal Failure:

   - Initiate fluids for hypotension (systolic BP less than 90 or MAP less than 65) or Lactate greater than or equal to 4

   Ideal body weight: 61.5 kg (135 lb 9.3 oz)

   ☑ Pharmacy Consult -STAT to calculate additional fluid to complete 15 mL/kg bolus using IBW
   Reason For Consult: to calculate additional fluid to complete 15 mL/kg bolus
   Sign
   ☐ For patient IBW 45.5—67 kg: lactated ringers infusion 15 mL/kg
   ☐ For patient IBW 45.5—67 kg: 0.9% sodium chloride infusion 15 mL/kg

Fig. 2. Sepsis order set for intravenous fluid management. * Indicates initiate fluids for hypotension (systolic BP less than 90 or MAP less than 65) or Lactate greater than or equal to 4.

pharmacist works with nursing to identify how much fluid had been given and then enters the rest of the needed fluid into the medication record for nursing to administer.

Adjustment to order sets ensured appropriate fluid resuscitation; however, providers still must document a volume status/tissue perfusion assessment within 6 hours if IVF resuscitation had been required. This is the final requirement to satisfy the bundle compliance. In 2022, CMS allowed for limited IVF resuscitation with very strict documentation requirements. Within our EMR, 2 smart phrases were created to allow the provider to pull in accurate and complete documentation to satisfy the volume status/tissue perfusion assessment and the limited IVF documentation. We were able to pull the BMI rule in as well. For example, if the BMI is greater than 30, use IBW and it joins it to the IVF Order. The IVF exception smart phrase includes exact wording and pick lists per CMS guidelines: IVF exception include hypotension, lactate 4 or greater, or septic shock, and the sepsis exception conditions included: concern for fluid overload, heart failure, renal failure, blood pressure responded to lesser volume, and a portion of the crystalloid fluid was administered as colloids. The amount of IVF boluses automatically pulls into the note for the last 12 hours (**Fig. 3**).

The order sets and smart phrases could only assist the provider so far. It was up to the provider to know when the 6-hour time out would occur or the case would fail. The SEP-1 core measure is a binary grading system (met/unmet) meaning that all actions

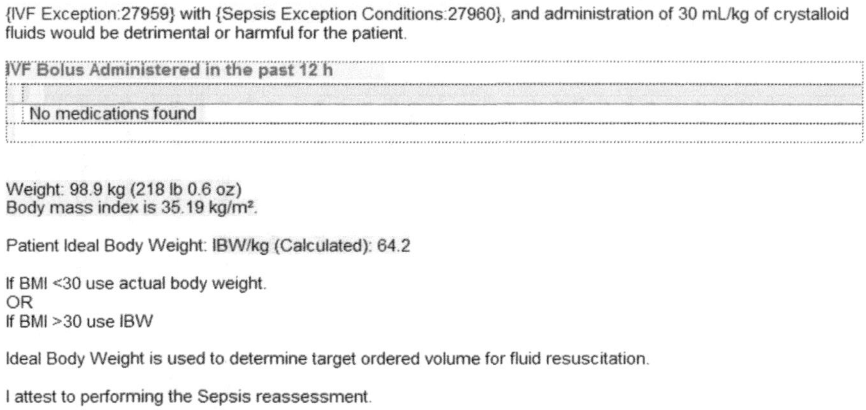

{IVF Exception:27959} with {Sepsis Exception Conditions:27960}, and administration of 30 mL/kg of crystalloid fluids would be detrimental or harmful for the patient.

IVF Bolus Administered in the past 12 h
No medications found

Weight: 98.9 kg (218 lb 0.6 oz)
Body mass index is 35.19 kg/m².

Patient Ideal Body Weight: IBW/kg (Calculated): 64.2

If BMI <30 use actual body weight.
OR
If BMI >30 use IBW

Ideal Body Weight is used to determine target ordered volume for fluid resuscitation.

I attest to performing the Sepsis reassessment.

Fig. 3. Sepsis smart phrase.

must be completed within the 3-hour and 6-hour time frame; if one element is missed, the case fails.

Process Improvement Project

A new workflow process to improve early recognition and sepsis core measure compliance

With the organization's ongoing commitment to abstract every case and the strict "all-or-nothing" measures mandated by CMS, the sepsis coordinator identified the need for 24/7 sepsis monitoring to improve early recognition, provider awareness, and prompt initiation of treatment.[14,15] The coordinator approached the nursing department with the idea to utilize the CMU, a remote unit that monitors telemetry and continuous video monitoring, to evaluate the BPA's 24/7. The Sepsis Coordinator collaborated with EMR analysts and clinical nurses in the CMU to create a customized sepsis BPA dashboard in the EMR. This dashboard supports the team in monitoring for early signs of sepsis aiding prompt recognition and treatment. A second dashboard checklist was customized to highlight the core measure components (**Fig. 4**). This new workflow improved sepsis compliance as well as improved patient outcomes:

- CMU reviews all sepsis BPAs that occur in the emergency department and inpatient areas.
- Evaluates each BPA for accurate sepsis data
  - *Severe sepsis criteria* = 2 SIRS, 1 one end-organ dysfunction + infection
  - *Septic shock criteria* = severe sepsis criteria + lactate 4 or greater and/or sustained hypotension
- CMU RN documentation in EMR for *probable sepsis* notification
- CMU RN contacts provider to evaluate patient for sepsis or septic shock
- Provider collaboration leads to utilization of specialized sepsis order sets with initiation of a sepsis timer
- If a provider declines sepsis criteria, a picklist within the EMR is selected to document the reason
- A customized sepsis checklist is used to monitor completed bundle measures (see **Fig. 4**).
  - Dashboard ensures all elements are occurring within the 3-hour and 6-hour timed requirements
  - All elements of the bundle are necessary to provide appropriate Sepsis Care as recommended by the SSC.

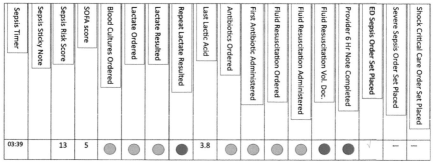

Fig. 4. Sepsis checklist.

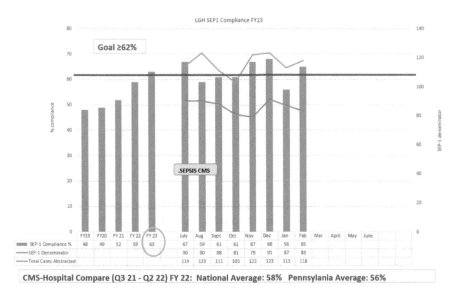

CMS-Hospital Compare (Q3 21 - Q2 22) FY 22: National Average: 58% Pennsylania Average: 56%

Fig. 5. CMS SEP-1 core measure compliance.

- CMU RN will contact provider/nurses for incomplete bundle elements
- CMU RN adds Sepsis clinical practice guidelines (CPG) to the care plan identifying patient as a sepsis survivor to all health-care team members across the continuum
  - Sepsis CPG identifies patient as sepsis survivor across the continuum
  - Sepsis CPG assists in communicating to the care management team needed Face-to-face–sepsis-after-care for postacute referrals
  - Sepsis CPG triggers the addition of sepsis survivor education to the EHR to assist the health-care teams to educate on important key elements of sepsis care

Collaboration with providers has led to improved use of specialized sepsis order sets, initiation of the sepsis timer, and utilization of a customized sepsis checklist allowing CMU nurses to monitor completed components required for SEP-1 compliance. Since fiscal year 2019, the organization has had a steady improvement in core measure compliance from 48% to 63% (current year to date [YTD] data), outperforming the national and state benchmarks (**Fig. 5**).

The organization continues to abstract and submit all case for overall awareness of compliance. Early recognition as well as targeted treatment has persistently allowed our mortality index to be less than 1.0 (compares the observed to expected mortality rates). A mortality ratio of more than 1.0 means the actual number of deaths exceeds the predicted number where as a ratio less than 1.0 means fewer patients died than expected. Ratios less than 1.0 suggest safer, higher quality care (**Fig. 6**).

Continuous Monitoring Unit Sepsis Case Study

0618: Triage: A 58-year-old woman arrives to emergency room complaining of left-sided abdominal and flank pain associated with nausea, vomiting, and shaking. She denies fever.

PMH included asthma, T2DM, hyperlipidemia (HLD), osteoarthritis, gastroesophageal reflux disease (GERD), and obesity. Surgical PMH: Gastric bypass

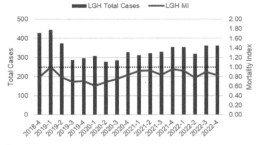

Fig. 6. Mortality index.

0619: 150/74 MAP 99 HR 103 RR 16 Temp 97.6 POX 98% Pain 7/10

0649: WBC 4.1 Glucose 159 Unable to produce urine for sample. NS 1000 mL bolus given. IV Zofran and tylenol given

1000: CT Abdomen completed, increase in pain. Morphine 4 mg IV given

1100: 76/52 MAP 60 HR 115 RR 16 POX 95%, hypotension d/t morphine, NS 1000 mL given

1110: 85/53 MAP 64 HR 115

1127: Sepsis BPA fires: HR 112 RR 24 with 2 hypotensive episodes; CMU RN pages provider and sepsis BPA ruled out; attributed to morphine.

1130: 87/51 MAP 63 HR 109, #3 NS 1000 mL given

1210: UA obtained, (+) sent for C&S

1215: CMU RN continues to monitor and notes (+) UA, calls provider for probable infection/sepsis. The provider was favoring a complicated urinary tract infection but after speaking with the CMU RN chose to launch the sepsis orders that escalated the care to stat and placed the patient on the sepsis dashboard.

1217: ED Sepsis Order set launched, Sepsis Timer started, Blood cultures ×2, Lactate w/repeat if greater than 2.0, Levaquin for probable urinary tract infection (UTI), IVF completed for weight 62.7; BMI 28 = 1890; 3 L NS completed

1315: Levaquin IV given

1327: 82/45 MAP 57 HR 135 RR 22 Temp 100.3 POX 97%; lactate 3.6; Levophed started

1401: Transferred to IVU for left hydronephrosis d/t obstructing stone, Perc nephrostomy tube placement.

1440: CMU RN contacts provider for sepsis reassessment evaluation and note completion.

1450: Admit to ICU

1740: Repeat Lactate 2.4, Next day: Levophed titrated off, morning laboratory work within normal limits, transferred to regular room.

Recently, a patient presented to the emergency department complaining of back pain, fevers, weakness, and her family noted that she was confused. Her laboratory work began to result and triggered the sepsis BPA for a slightly elevated creatinine and lactate (2 laboratory results that indicate organ dysfunction). The CMU RN noted that the urine analysis was positive and contacted the provider. The provider was favoring a complicated urinary tract infection but after collaborating with the CMU RN, the provider chose to launch the sepsis orders, which escalated the care to stat and placed the patient on the sepsis dashboard allowing for close oversight by the CMU RN. With close monitoring, the CMU RN was able to monitor for possible deterioration. The patient soon developed hypotension and the CMU RN and pharmacist were able to ensure that all interventions were completed successfully within the 3-hour and 6-hour core measure bundle. The patient's creatinine and lactate quickly returned to normal due to effective source control, antibiotic administration, and fluid resuscitation. The patient was successfully discharged without any other complications. Launching the sepsis CPG to the care plan allowed awareness to all team members that this patient was a sepsis survivor. Care management coordinated home health for close follow-up at discharge. Follow-up appointments to the primary care provider and urology were made before discharge to support a smooth transition of care back to home. Sepsis education was preloaded to the after visit summary, which included information for monitoring and prevention of sepsis as well as a clinical pathway for daily activities to improve patient outcomes. This process relies on nursing, providers, and pharmacy completing real-time communication and collaboration. If one team member does not complete their part, the process falls apart. The success of this new workflow has been attributed to the importance of team dedication to communication and collaboration for early interventions to meet SSC recommendations.

CLINICS CARE POINTS: *EVIDENCE-BASED PEARLS*

- Early sepsis identification leads to rapid intervention and reduced mortality.
- Older adults can have atypical signs and symptoms of sepsis.
- Fluid resuscitation of at least 30 mL/kg is essential to restore circulating volume for most patients in septic shock.
- Exception to the rule for patients that may have a need to limit fluid resuscitation: end-stage renal disease, congestive heart failure, and other possible comorbid conditions.
- Utilization of sepsis order sets based on SCC recommendations improves patient outcomes.

INITIATIVES TO REDUCE READMISSIONS

According to Sepsis Alliance, "the average cost per hospital stay is double the average cost per stay across all other conditions. And, sepsis is the primary cause of readmissions to the hospital, costing more than 3.5 billion each year."[16] Early in 2020, our organization recognized the need for better understanding of all sepsis readmissions. An A3, a structured problem solving and continuous improvement approach, was instituted. The first step was to understand why patients returned to the hospital. Interviews were conducted and feedback highlighted a lack of understanding of the sepsis diagnosis, the importance of follow-up with the primary provider, and steps to prevent further infections. Based on the A3 findings, the CMU workflow was amended to include loading the Sepsis Clinical Practice Guideline to the Care Plan in the EMR. This allows disciplines to see sepsis as a primary focus escalating it above the infection. Sepsis as a primary focus heightens awareness of organ dysfunction putting the patient at an increased risk for complications. This prompts sepsis after care education to be addressed before discharge and is added to the after visit summary. Education is focused on the following topics:

- Sepsis prevention
- Time matters
- Life after sepsis
- Recovery steps

In the past year, our organization has partnered with the Penn School of Nursing in a multisite hybrid implementation science study called I-TRANSFER project

(Improving TRansitions ANd outcomeS oF sEpsis suRvivors) (Grant #: 2R01NR016014-03). The focus of the study is to implement an evidence-based protocol for timely home health nursing visits (2 visits within 7 days of discharge with the start of care being within 2 days of hospital discharge) and an outpatient provider visit by day 7. In a national comparative effectiveness study, sepsis survivors who received this pattern of care had readmission rates 7% lower than those without timely postacute attention. This study has promoted improved documentation of sepsis survivors in the discharge summary. Referral documents have increased referrals to home health care, which have improved communication between the care management team and home health care liaisons. This has increased attention to patient and caregiver education, and has reinforced the need to make the outpatient appointment before hospital discharge.

Our organization is currently incorporating the I-TRANSFER project. The Sepsis CPG along with the sepsis diagnosis assists in communication to the care management team to reach out to providers to order home health and telehealth remote monitoring. The organization's home health agency, with the awareness of a sepsis diagnosis, initiates follow-up within 24 to 48 hours of discharge and adds telehealth for close monitoring. The home health agency educates the patient and caregiver on the telemedicine platform, which will screen the patient's daily vital signs and uses a questionnaire to note changes in status for possible escalation of care to the primary care provider. In keeping with the I-TRANSFER protocol, the home health RN will start home health within 2 days and provide at least 2 visits in the first week and will promote a primary care visit within 7 days of discharge. A Personal Sepsis Pathway survivor tool has been created and provided to patients and home health caregivers to monitor recovery progression.

COMPONENTS OF A PERSONAL SEPSIS PATHWAY ASSESSMENT TOOL FOR SEPSIS SURVIVORS

- Follow-up with primary care provider within 1 week
- Daily morning weight
- Monitor temperature, pain, and changes in wounds daily
- Track mood and energy
- Monitor for urine output every 8 hours
- Nutrition: well-balanced diet and fluid intake per provider order
- Increase activity as able
- Discuss goals and health-care wishes with family and provider

Preliminary results for this project have shown a significant impact on readmission for sepsis survivors enrolled with our I-TRANSFER agency (**Fig. 7**).

DISCUSSION: *ONGOING OPPORTUNITIES*

- Continuing provider education on early recognition and treatment to prevent septic shock
- Provider support for documentation requirements for CMS compliance
- Continuing RN recruitment to support CMU 24/7
- Branch out to other home health agencies to incorporate the I-TRANSFER components
- Advanced care planning conversations with patients and families
- Persistent dedication to building team collaboration to promote improvements and innovative methods, improve early recognition

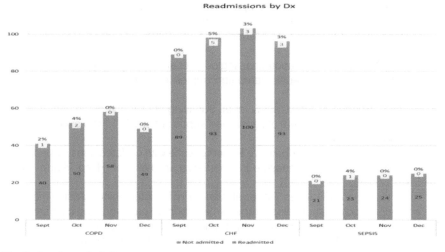

Fig. 7. Sepsis readmissions.

Summary

The commitment from the organization to submit all cases to CMS provided opportunities and challenges for the sepsis coordinator to meet program goals. The new workflow process project with CMU supports a platform to bring evidence-based care to patients vital for positive outcomes. The collaborative work with providers, pharmacists, nursing department, case management, and the organization's home health agency continues to improve SEP-1 compliance and transition of care to reduce readmissions.

DISCLOSURE

The I-TRANSFER study is supported by the National Institute of Nursing Research [NINR] grant number 2R01NR016014-03. The content is solely the responsibility of the authors and does not necessarily represent the official views of the National Institutes of Health.

REFERENCES

1. Sepsis fact sheet - sepsis alliance. Available at: https://cdn.sepsis.org/wp-content/uploads/2018/08/Sepsis-Fact-Sheet-2018-LA-8_1_182.pdf. Accessed December 11, 2022.
2. What is sepsis? Centers for Disease Control and Prevention. Available at: https://www.cdc.gov/sepsis/what-is-sepsis.html. Published August 9, 2022. Accessed November 31, 2022.
3. Global report on the epidemiology and burden of sepsis: Current evidence, identifying gaps and future directions. World Health Organization. Available at: https://who.int/publications/i/item/9789240010789. Published September 9, 2020. Accessed November 31, 2022.
4. Rowe TA, McKoy JM. Sepsis in Older Adults. Infect Dis Clin North Am 2017;31(4): 731–42.
5. The SEP-1 Measure: What is it, and how does it impact sepsis patients & their families. Available at: https://www.sepsis.org/news/the-sep-1-measure-what-is-

it-and-how-does-it-impact-sepsis-patients-their-families/#: ~ :text=%E2%80%
9CSEP%2D1%E2%80%9D%20is%20shorthand,early%20intervention%20with%
20lifesaving%20therapies. Published June 22, 2021. Accessed December 11,
2022.

6. Schorr CA, Seckel MA, Papathanassoglou E, et al. Nursing implications of the updated 2021 surviving sepsis campaign guidelines. Am J Crit Care 2022;31(4):
329–36.

7. Evans L, Rhodes A, Alhazzani W, et al. Surviving sepsis campaign: international
guidelines for management of sepsis and septic shock 2021. Intensive Care Med
2021;47:1181–247.

8. Ramsdell TH, Smith AN, Kerkhove E. Compliance with updated sepsis bundles to
meet new sepsis core measure in a tertiary care hospital. Hosp Pharm 2017;
52(3):177–86.

9. Rhee C, Brown SR, Jones TM, et al. Variability in determining sepsis time zero
and bundle compliance rates for the centers for medicare and medicaid services
SEP-1 measure. Infect Control Hosp Epidemiol 2018;39(8):994–6.

10. Rhee C, Filbin MR, Massaro AF, et al. Compliance with the national SEP-1 quality
measure and association with sepsis outcomes: a multicenter retrospective
cohort study. Crit Care Med 2018;46(10):1585–91.

11. Vincent JL. The clinical challenge of sepsis identification and monitoring. PLoS
Med 2016;13(5):e1002022.

12. Sinapidis D, Kosmas V, Vittoros V, et al. Progression into sepsis: an individualized
process varying by the interaction of comorbidities with the underlying infection.
BMC Infect Dis 2018;18(1):242.

13. Truong T-TN, Dunn AS, McCardle K, et al. Adherence to fluid resuscitation guidelines and outcomes in patients with septic shock: reassessing the "one-size-fits-
all" approach. J Crit Care 2019;51:94–8.

14. Li Q, Wang J, Liu G, et al. Prompt admission to intensive care is associated with
improved survival in patients with severe sepsis and/or septic shock. J Int Med
Res 2018;46(10):4071–81.

15. Hu B, Xiang H, Dong Y, et al. Timeline of sepsis bundle component completion
and its association with Septic Shock Outcomes. J Crit Care 2020;60:143–51.

16. What is sepsis. Sepsis Alliance. Available at: https://www.sepsis.org/sepsis-
basics/what-is-sepsis/. Published February 7, 2023. Accessed January 21, 2023.

An Interprofessional Precision Health Model for Assessment of Caregiver Impact on Polypharmacy in Elderly Intensive Care Unit Patients

A Team-Based Proposal

Debbra Pogue, PhD, APRN, ACNS-BC, CCRN-K, CHSE[a],*,
Mary O'Keefe, JD, PhD, APRN, CNS P/MH, LPC, FAAN[b]

KEYWORDS

- Interprofessional • Caregiver • Elderly • Critical care • Polypharmacy
- Precision medicine • Precision health • Pharmacogenomics

KEY POINTS

- The interprofessional approach may empower informal caregivers and family members.
- Competence in precision health concepts is needed to optimize application to care of the elderly.
- Nurses have skills to develop, collaborate, and conduct innovative research.

INTRODUCTION

Precision health is defined as both the treatment and prevention methods that encompass unique attributes and associated variability of each patient.[1–3] Precision health has been referred to as individualized medicine and was formerly known as precision medicine but now carries a broader moniker for increased inclusivity.[4] Precision health is health care customized to the patient. It is such a broad and multifaceted initiative that requires the engagement and participation of interprofessional health care professionals for successful acquisition and usage of data. The topic of precision health is interprofessional and can include physicians, nurses, social workers, engineers, information technologists, biostatisticians, and information technology analysts. There has

[a] Our Lady of the Lake Regional Medical Center, 5246 Brittany Drive, Baton Rouge, LA 70808, USA; [b] University of Texas Medical Branch at Galveston, Room 4.Room 4.231, Route 1132301 University Boulevard, Galveston, TX 77555-1029
* Corresponding author. 5246 Brittany Drive, Baton Rouge, LA 70808.
E-mail address: dpogue@lsuhsc.edu

Crit Care Nurs Clin N Am 35 (2023) 425–451
https://doi.org/10.1016/j.cnc.2023.07.001
0899-5885/23/© 2023 Elsevier Inc. All rights reserved.

ccnursing.theclinics.com

been success in the application of precision health in several fields such as oncology and pharmacogenetics.[5–8]

BACKGROUND

The Precision Medicine Initiative (PMI) was created in 2015, with the allocation of 215 million dollars to health efforts by former President Barack Obama.[3,9] For the PMI, community databases, public databases, and electronic health records (EHR) are important components for data classification and data collection. Interoperability between databases is needed for full access to data for PMI. The goals and objectives of precision health are to improve and perpetuate optimal health and reduce health care costs. These objectives are met by studying and acknowledging the impact of several factors including genetic, environmental, pharmacogenomic, behavioral, and social factors.[7] In addition, data may be used to predict outcomes in specific populations or groups. Moreover, precision health includes the integration of health information technology (HIT) into the delivery and management of health care.[4] HIT remains a critical branch of precision health for access, screening, point-of-care monitoring, tracking, and management of various health disparities affecting diverse populations. Within the EHR, a greater emphasis is now placed on understanding the social determinants of health (SDoH). Because of the potential for multiple areas of impact, precision health may serve as a structural model for many initiatives. Meaningful use of the data should be the responsibility of medicine, nursing, pharmacy, and partner academic health institutions.[4,10]

Elderly patients have been reported as the largest group of patients treated in the intensive care units (ICUs).[11] They are a vulnerable group due to aging organ systems, specifically the neurologic, hepatic, and renal system, and their ability to metabolize and excrete drugs. Much as screening is performed to assess SDoH, screening for events related to polypharmacy on admission and at discharge should be standard.

In the United States, there are more than 65.7 million informal caregivers.[3] The informal caregivers or family members often accompany patients to multiple appointments to see various specialty providers. In addition, in situations where mentation is limited due to cognitive decline, medications, and health conditions, the informal caregiver or family member is often the recipient of discharge instructions.

Interprofessional team-based care can positively affect adverse reactions related to polypharmacy in the critically ill elderly patient. Key team members such as the physicians, nurses, pharmacists, respiratory care technicians, and several others can engage the informal caregiver or family member at any point during the hospitalization and capture vital information and/or provide education on care for the impaired or incapacitated patient. Strong interprofessional teams facilitate sharing of information, coordination, and follow-up and eliminate hierarchical practices.[12,13] Health care teams realize that if their interventions and best practices do not extend into the community and/or patient's homes, health care team efforts may be futile, can result in subsequent readmissions, and can be a cyclical failure to prevent injury and harm.[4] The suboptimal culture of pharmacologic safety may also result in increased costs due to extended length of stay and exacerbations in chronic conditions.[14] It has been well documented that polypharmacy in the critically ill patient may affect the patient once discharged.[6,15] For example, according to AHRQ's Chartbook on Patient Safety, 11.7% of non-Hispanic black patients who received hypoglycemic agents experienced adverse reactions related to the agent[16] in stark contrast to the 4.3% of non-Hispanic white patients.[17] An additional example of suboptimal pharmacologic safety is when critical care nurses report mixed feelings about the efficacy, harm, and lingering effects of tight or aggressive glycemic control in critically ill patients and note multiple changes and recommendations to sliding scale insulin protocols based on their objective assessment data.[18]

An example of the predictive nature of genome profiling is Hector Wong's Genomics of Pediatric Septic Shock. The study found 3 subclasses (endotype A, B, and C). Endotype A consisted of younger patients with a higher mortality risk and higher illness severity. As a result, these patients responded differently to corticosteroid therapy, commonly used in sepsis treatment.[19] The AHRQ's Chartbook on Patient Safety further indicated that providers do not explain things in ways that patients understand, resulting in varied benchmark projections for success across racial strata.

Pharmacogenomics is gradually being used to relate biomarkers, genetic variants, and drug information relative to polymorphisms to poorly represented minority and ethnic groups.[7,20] Perhaps pharmacogenomics research may shed light as to why the differences in response to insulin dose adjustments vary across ethnic groups. There are already several cases in which metabolic uptake of certain drugs is erratic due to enzymes such as CYP450 and receptors in persons of African American/Black descent.[7]

IMPORTANCE OF PRECISION HEALTH TO NURSING SCIENCE

Precision health is important to nursing science because nurses are essential caregivers and provide care across the continuum. Nurses play an active role in assessing, diagnosing, providing interventions, evaluating, and recommending referrals as part of the interprofessional team. As nursing scientists, it is important to study the population's SDoH to design, customize, and adapt appropriate care. The National Institutes of Nursing Research (NINR) and the National Institutes of Health (NIH) are both entities that encourage advanced research education and opportunities for nurses to affect the populations they serve.[3] Symptom science and self-reporting are encouraged in patients. Symptom science is a branch of research using basic (patient reported), clinical (assessment or laboratory results/diagnostics), or translational (application) research to gain an understanding of symptom presentation as well as how it is affected by the environment. Symptom science also studies the characteristics and presentations of symptoms, such as whether they exist in clusters and how it affects outcomes of physical and mental health.[5,10] Precision health and symptom science present opportunities for nurses to take a proactive stance in the management of health disparities through research, data collection, data analysis, and dissemination as members of the interprofessional health care team. Nurse researchers, by virtue of their positions, are in a role that may positively contribute to the nursing body of knowledge and precision health data.

An interprofessional model is suggested because elderly patients accounted for 27.8 million hospital admissions from 1996 to 2010.[11] Elderly patients account for approximately half of the critical care admissions due to inappropriate prescriptions.[15] Falls and complications of multiple comorbidities are additional reasons for admission. As such, older patient admissions often result in the need for multiple services to address each condition. For example, health care encounters with older adults may involve emergency medicine, internal medicine, cardiology or renal, and even orthopedics if fractures occur. These admissions may be further complicated due to exacerbation in chronic diseases or missed routine follow-ups that increased exponentially during the intra- and post-COVID-19 pandemic.[21] In the ICU, patients may experience dementia or delirium and may not understand changes that were made in their prescription regimens and may fail to communicate changes to other providers they subsequently visit on discharge. Even more concerning is the fact that some patients are discharged from the ICU on an inappropriate medication that may contribute to adverse reactions. A key point is that critical care nurses may rely heavily on caregivers or family members to provide information or serve as a resource during the hospitalization of the elderly patient.[22] The same is true on discharge.

PURPOSE

The purpose of this literature review is to define the concept of precision health and review the evidence describing its use as an interprofessional model for assessing caregiver impact on polypharmacy in elderly ICU patients. This article also discusses literature describing an ICU-focused interprofessional precision health model for assessment of caregiver impact on polypharmacy in elderly ICU patients. The overarching goal is to determine the potential for improvement in hospital admission rates and length of stay due to polypharmacy by using the interprofessional precision health care model for elderly patients. In addition, information concerning oversight and facilitation of the medication regimen by the informal caregivers of dependent and independent seniors may provide information to warrant deprescription and reduce risk and improve quality of life.

THE RESEARCH QUESTIONS

The research question guiding the literature review was "How can an interprofessional precision health model be utilized for the assessment of provider impact on polypharmacy of critically ill elderly patients?" After conducting a literature review, the answers to the following 2-fold research questions are provided.

1. Will an interprofessional precision health model improve provider impact on the medication regimen for critically ill elderly patients?
2. Will an interprofessional precision health model decrease the number of adverse drug-related events related to polypharmacy in the critically ill elderly patients?

SEARCH STRATEGIES

Databases searched included CINAHL, Cochrane Library, EBSCOhost, Genomic Data Commons, OVID PubMed, ScienceDirect, and Scopus. Genomic Data Commons was selected because genomics is a subheading of one of the many arms of precision health and oncologic impact is an important study area. The NIH RePORTER was selected to examine other potential sources of data for precision health that has been previously funded by NIH. Delimiters were peer-reviewed journals, primary sources, and those written in the English language published between 2013 and 2023. Keywords used were precision health, precision medicine, precision health initiative, model, precision health model, caregiver assessment, model, elderly, critical care, interprofessional, caregivers, and informal caregivers. The review yielded 29 studies meeting inclusion criteria: 1 systematic review, 13 literature reviews, 3 randomized controlled trials, 2 opinion/editorial reviews, 1 pilot study, 1 observational, 1 retrospective cohort study, 2 quantitative, 1 prospective cohort study, 1 grounded phenomenology, 1 integrative review, 1 narrative review, 1 review and perspective, and several other types embedded within the literature reviews (**Table 1**; PRISMA Diagram).

Table 1
The integrated review table summarizes and provides an overview of selected studies

No.	Author/s Date	Research Question	Design & Method	Population Sample (Size, Type)	Data Collection/ Instruments	Analysis	Findings	Strengths	Limitations	Conclusion	Implications (Take Home Message)
1	Akroute & Bondas,[22] 2016	What are CCNs' experiences with relatives of elderly patients >80 y?	Grounded Phenomenology Interpretive Qualitative Research	6 CCNs	Semistructured personal interviews	Graneheim & Lundman method, emerging themes	CCNs' feelings were ambivalent. Relatives were viewed as resources or seen as challenges	Qualitative studies offer understanding of behavior and worldview, data were rich	Small sample size of 6 nurses Single clinical setting Male to female ratio	CCN's experiences were mixed	Communication, education, reflection, and structured organization may improve holistic family nursing for elderly patients
2	Ashley,[23] 2015	N/A	Opinion	Not specified	Literature review	Summary	The PMI may be useful in fine-tuning clinical research. Many drugs are approved; however, only a small amount of study participants drive study results when data are scrutinized based on number needed to treat (NNT)	Gave relatable examples of PM in current use, how genomic sequencing is used and use of genetic information for prescribing	Did not list details of studies mentioned nor type of study (that is, RCT vs quasi-experimental)	Prevention and oncology advancements via pharmacogenomic study will be promising areas in the future	Prevention is an area that has promise.
3	Bosen et al,[12] 2015	What are emerging roles for telemedicine & smart technology in dementia care?	Literature review (qualitative studies)	N/A	Literature review	Summary	Technology must be easy to use, may benefit patient and caregiver, especially GPS tracking	Utilization of both quantitative and qualitative data	Was not a systemic review	Technology has a beneficial place in home care to assist both patients living with dementia and their caregivers	Technology may reduce the caregiver burden and improve quality of life; however, future research is needed to determine cost-effectiveness.
4	Cacchione,[9] 2016	What is the role of nursing in Precision Medicine?	Editorial	Not specified	Literature Review	Summary	Interprofessional partnerships are encouraged to manage data collected for precision health	Succinct listing of potential benefits of precision medicine and the role nursing may play in achieving success	No specification of types of studies reviewed (ie, RCTs, quasi-experimental studies, and so on)	No single discipline can facilitate the analysis needed for precision medicine, thus necessitating an interprofessional approach.	Precision medicine and nursing can symbiotically create positive outcomes in several areas such as cancer and other areas of research.
5	Chi & Demiris,[24] 2014	What telehealth tools exist to support family caregivers?	Systematic Review (52 experimental studies—19	Varied: 20 articles included more than 100 participants, 13 included	Systematic literature review	Two-researcher analysis using Oxford Center for Evidence-	Use of telehealth for caregivers included education, consultation,	Level of evidence was high to medium per Oxford Center for	Several studies had a low level of evidence strength	Most of the studies indicated outcome improvement satisfaction with telehealth	Technology may be instrumental in achieving positive outcomes and improve caregiver ability to manage patients and benefit from

(continued on next page)

Table 1 *(continued)*

No.	Author/s Date	Research Question	Design & Method	Population Sample (Size, Type)	Data Collection/ Instruments	Analysis	Findings	Strengths	Limitations	Conclusion	Implications (Take Home Message)
			RCTs, 33 non-RCT (pilot, feasibility, comparison, quasi-experimental, and pretest/ posttest design), 11 evaluation studies, 1 case study, one secondary analysis.	50–100 participants, 25 included 10–50 participants, and 7 articles included <10 participants		Based Medicine framework	and psychiatric or behavioral health therapy	Evidence-based Medicine framework			enhanced communication with health care providers
6	Collins, Varmus,[1] 2015	What are the main initiatives of precision medicine?	Review & perspective	N/A	Literature review	Summary	Plan for assembly of a 1 million participant cohort for longitudinal study	Studies to be assembled from current NIH-funded studies is an excellent use of current resources already in place	Did not provide detail or provide multiple types of studies used to collect information. Focused on oncology studies as part of near-term goals.	Two broad initiatives: near-term focus on cancer, long-term aim to generate knowledge to health & disease	Data collection for this initiative may provide pharmacogenetic insight for drug targeting
7	Fänge AM et al. 2017	What is the efficacy of an innovative technological intervention in persons living with dementia and the primary informal caregivers?	RCT	Persons living with dementia, 320 dyads (640 persons total) including caregivers	SPIRIT checklist Swedish National Health Survey, IADL (Instrumental Activities of Daily Living), RUD Questionnaire	Standard protocol and checklist	Interventions to support caregiver may decrease use of certain antipsychotic medications	Use of RCTs and large sample size	Did not provide focus or detail on methods to assist with polypharmacy	Success demonstrated in easing caregiver burden with integrated home and monitoring. Reduction in caregiver burden and anxiety may translate to polypharmacy and prescription regimen, especially through reporting of adverse events.	Dementia rates will triple by 2050, and informal caregivers are increasing. Data collection via precision health and technology may ease caregiver and health care cost burden, especially with regard to drug utilization.
8	Fangonil-Gagalang E, Schultz MA 2021	What is the method to introduce precision health into baccalaureate nursing curriculum?	Pilot study	Small urban nursing college	5-item survey	5 semesters pos-timplementation	Nursing students are introduced to research and the scientific process. Precision health can be easily integrated into that education.	Pilot study with evaluation via survey	Small sample size.	Stepwise	Nurse educators should encourage introduction of precision health terminology and concepts in nursing curriculum

#	Author, Year	Research Question	Study Design	Sample	Literature/Tools	Proposed/Summary	Findings	Study Types	Limitations	Conclusion	Recommendations
9	Fujita et al,[25] 2023	What are the challenges in achieving precision medicine in polypharmacy?	Narrative review (qualitative, systematic review, observational, interventional studies, RCTs, miscellaneous clinical trials)	Young, old male mice, middle-aged mice, female mice at various ages and levels of polypharmacy	STOPP, START, CDSS, PRISCUS list, SENATOR, G-MEDSS, DBI, BEERS	Proposed precision medicine to be incorporated into medication review for patients with polypharmacy	There are several tools to monitor and assess polypharmacy and intervene where necessary. Phenotypic data have resulted in published guidelines on drug adjustment based on genetic tests. Recommended to operationalize and integrate pharmacogenomics into physician and pharmacy workflow.	Multiple studies and designs and methods, experimental groups	There was a reported lack of data on the effect of sex and gender on polypharmacy, thus limiting generalizability of results.	Precision medicine is important in drug-gene, drug-disease, and drug-food interactions. By considering drug metabolism in the elderly due to aging, adverse effects may be minimized.	Recommendation to incorporate the technological framework associated with precision medicine. Drug and geriatric syndrome interactions (falls, frailty, and confusion) are more likely in the presence of polypharmacy.
10	Gameiro et al,[10] 2018	In What Ways Can Precision Medicine Change the Way We Think About Healthcare?	Literature Review (Multiple experimental studies referenced)	Varies Not Specified	Literature Review (Multiple references for experimental studies cited)	Summary	Four Ps of precision medicine: prediction, prevention, participation, personalization	Consisted of multiple types of reference studies per in-text and bibliographical references.	No table summarizing types of literature, findings, and literature used	Precision medicine provides the promise of personalized treatment and multiple areas of impact but presents challenges such as the ethical issues involved with the collection and access to data in the repository.	Precision medicine opens possibilities for technological advances and an increased call for collaboration among interprofessional team members including the patients to improve biomedical outcomes and science. It is important to continue to facilitate a global approach from other countries with regard to data collection.
11	Hickey et al,[2] 2019	How can precision health be used to advance symptom science & self-management science?	Literature Review Case Study of NINR P30 Centers of Excellence	Multiple NINR P20 and P30 Centers of Excellence	NSPH Model requires the integral nursing leadership to ensure measurement, describe phenotype, describe genotype and the targeted creation of the intervention via design, delivery, and discovery	Table outlining symptom foci, exemplars of self-management & contributions and future impact on precision health	Pain, sleep, and cognition were among some of the most prevalent symptom foci	Multiple geographic research sites NINR P20/P30 Centers of Excellence selected	Multiple practice areas represented demonstrating promising use of precision health; however, only one study in all mentioned interprofessional team usage of precision health	The NSPH model of 4 components of precision health can advance symptom science. It is imperative to approach the task from the goal of prevention as well as curing or treating disease processes.	Continue the advancement of symptom science successfully with precision health, education on genomics, and training incorporated into programs and grants. Ensure that precision health transitions from research into the practice of population health.

(continued on next page)

Table 1
(continued)

No.	Author/s Date	Research Question	Design & Method	Population Sample (Size, Type)	Data Collection/ Instruments	Analysis	Findings	Strengths	Limitations	Conclusion	Implications (Take Home Message)
12	Hull,[3] 2018	Describe nursing's readiness for precision health	Literature review	N/A	Literature review	The article discusses opportunities for supporting nurses and interprofessional care teams to add an additional layer of implementation of precision health into current care practices through symptom science, pharmacogenomics, social and behavioral health practices	There are several opportunities in existence to use symptom science, pharmacogenomic science from a social and health care standpoint to address disease processes benefitting from symptom science interventions.	The authors advocate for nurse managers to take an increase in role and for the advancement of nursing researchers. Nurses are asked to focus their nursing care on where patients work, play, and live. Subsequently, the studies revealed several nurse-led models created to address patients with significant health care cost burdens. Publication also mentioned family caregivers.	Did not specify or distinguish many interprofessional studies although mentioned in the article.	Nurses require support in leveraging knowledge, decision support tools, and EHRs to use data for symptom science and pharmacogenomics. Publication was one of the few articles to mention the inclusion of family caregivers in addition to social and behavioral factors for consideration when using precision health.	The role of nurse managers will evolve to support and prepare nurses. Nurse leadership will be integral in integration of symptom science and individualized care.
13	Javier et al,[4] 2020	How accurate is race and ethnicity as indicated by the VHA common data model? How useful is the classification schema at prioritizing ethnicity for disparities work?	Quantitative	VHA patients N = 9176 Hispanic/ Latino = 1415 Non-Hispanic Black = 2455 Non-Hispanic White = 5306	Patient Engagement Survey ("if, then" statements in 3 classification schemas) in SAS version 9.4	All agreement values were >80% using 3 classification schemas	Schema 1 had highest values across all indicators for hispanic/latino individuals compared with Schema 2/3. Schema 3 showed correct prediction only 56% of the time. In Schema 2 & 3 the model reliably classified	Agreement values were 80% or greater indicating reliability. Multiple race and ethnicities were represented.	Population was limited to veterans. No indication for gender was provided. Geographic location was not available from this article.	The model accurately represented the ethnic and racial makeup of the large sample of veterans when self-reported Hispanic/Latino ethnicity is prioritized over race.	It is important to ensure the accuracy of the data used from repositories and to ensure that language is standardized to ensure accuracy for disparity work.

14	Karolak et al,[5] 2018	What is the role mathematical models play in precision medicine and what are the quantitative frameworks that exist to complement experimental studies?	Literature review (discussing multiple experimental models)	Various mathematical models (inclusive of 3-d models, 2-d hexagonal cellular automaton, de novo, in vitro, in silico, in vivo, multicellular spheroid)	Mathematical computation and experimental observations	Analysis showed that only 10% of phenotypic heterogeneity was found in some biopsies, indicating that some treatments were ineffective in treating tumors due to lack of targeted genetic material	There were a few models that able to aid in the design of combination therapies and reducing toxicity.	Focus was placed on single DNA bases, which is paramount for personalized studies. The studies also looked at the interactions between the cells and microenvironments. Experimental study was used.		Studies require collaboration between multiple interdisciplinary groups for effective collection of data used.	Multiple models exist for cancer-related treatment. Each model has a unique approach and benefit based on the type of cancer diagnosis.	The application of mathematical models to cancer treatment would benefit from the inclusion of some of the intracellular, cellular, and intercellular-scale specifications.
15	Kluwe et al,[20] 2020	What are the challenges for model-informed precision dosing (MIPD)?	Literature review	Not specified	Literature review	There are multiple opportunities for both investigational and previously approved drugs to benefit from MIPD. There is also value in genetic and biomarker research as well as clinical care, however, clinical curriculum changes are needed for both physicians and pharmaceutical educational programs	Several aspects were listed in which MIPD may be beneficial in addition to drug development and regulation. The review presented several challenges as well as opportunities.	The review offered a very organized table of aspects and/or challenges and supporting information as well as recommendations and future implications.		Although the investigators mention collaboration, physicians and pharmacists are mentioned; however, nursing is excluded from this article. There is little mention of nursing even with regard to future opportunities. There is opportunity to foster complete interdisciplinary collaboration.	Data collection via mobile devices and other tools is increasing. Decision-making tools and MIPD can help to individualize medication prescription rather than a broad application. The future is to involve pharmaceutical companies and agencies that regulate pharmacotherapeutics.	To improve the usage of MIPD the investigators propose standardization of terminology among interprofessional disciplines to foster collaboration. They also make the call for multistakeholder collaboration to aid drug development from the development stage to bedside interventions and purport the need to evaluate, validate, and note the value of MIPD.
16	Mahoney MR, Asch SM.	What is the effect on a human-wide	Quantitative, experimental	50 patients (targeting	Surveys, genetic screening.	Using screening results and	The use of technology and	Three-fold operative to	11% to 12% of non-Hispanic white and 7% to 13% of non-Hispanic black individuals from self-report data.	Small sample size, however, varies	Both patient and provider interest in genetic testing aided with	The human-wide project is an example of how technology and assistive

(continued on next page)

Table 1
(continued)

No.	Author/s Date	Research Question	Design & Method	Population Sample (Size, Type)	Data Collection/ Instruments	Analysis	Findings	Strengths	Limitations	Conclusion	Implications (Take Home Message)
	Humanwide 2019	demonstration in building health care plans?		cancer and cardiovascular disease).	wearables, health assessments and wellness coaching	predictive analytics	devices such as bluetooth-enabled scales, glucometers, blood pressure cuffs, pedometers, and so on coupled with genetic information allowed physicians to detect poor control and prevent complications much earlier than in the absence of the tools.	predict & prevent disease more precisely and to cure more precisely. Also implemented prescribing practice of drug-gene reaction.	in ethnic, racial, genetic, and age groups as well as medical condition	enrollment. The investigators mention enhanced education on genetic screening and conditions was helpful among primary care patients and providers although which providers was not specified.	devices can result in early screening, early treatment, and early prescriptive therapy being provided. The prescriptive therapy can further be precisely selected based on genetic makeup to customize the dosage using pharmacogenetic testing with regard to gene-drug reaction. The patient-centered approach is but one enhancement to care.
17	Majumder et al,[6] 2017	What are the research challenges and advances for smart homes for the elderly?	Literature review	N/A	Literature review (multiple references from several studies cited)	The number of persons living with chronic diseases (heart disease, diabetes, obesity, and asthma) is increasing. Most of the chronic diseases are costly but can be prevented especially in the rapidly increasing elderly population.	In addition to e-health, M-health is available and summarizes the use of mobile device technology and mobile monitoring. Telemedicine also provides support for remote health care and has demonstrated decreases in mortality.	The advances mentioned in the article include electronic sharing of data with shared services such as caregivers, EMS, central station, hospitals, and physician's offices. The investigators offer a 4-layer approach to the development of a smart home. Multiple methods of remote health monitoring including vital signs, smart beds, and detecting falls is	Artificial intelligence (AI) is discussed minimally, especially its relationship to automated drug delivery. AI can also be used to monitor environmental cues and detect hazards such as gas leaks or smoke. Interoperability is a concern among the many types of devices and lack of standardization. The number of studies based in the United States was limited in comparison to the global studies from around the world.	Although there is the ever present concern for security and privacy in sharing and handling data, remote monitoring options remain a promising tool in treating the elderly in their own environments. The advancement in remote monitoring leads to low-power, low-cost tools to assist elderly patients.	The smart home is a technological advance that offers several health services to the patients' homes. Seamless operation of the many facets of remote health care delivery rely on the internet and integrations with biomedical data collection and storage. More research is needed to purposefully implement these initiatives with minimal interruption and consistent delivery without delay.

offered in this article.

#	Study	Research question	Design	Sample	Instruments / Analysis	Builds on	Relevance	Trial status	Conclusions	Implications
18	Malmgren Fänge et al.,[26] 2017; Morgan et al.,[27] 2017	What is the effect of information and communication technology on caregiver burden among caregivers of people living with dementia?	RCT duration 12 mo	320 dyads of persons living with dementia and their informal caregivers. Recruited from a memory clinic 160 per study arm with statistical power of 0.8% and 20% drop out rate, resulting in 128 dyads per each arm of study (experimental and control)	Home monitoring kit questionnaire (12-section) Resource Utilization in Dementia (RUD) Quality of Life in Alzheimer's Disease (QOL-AD) Falls Efficacy Scale-International (FES-I) European quality of life EuroQol 5D-3L Hospital Anxiety & Depression Scale (HADS) Zarit Burden Inventory (ZBI) Instrumental Activities of Daily Living (IADL) Home visits (at enrollment, 3 mo & 12 mo) following installation of information and communication & technology (ICT) kit	First RCT exploring the ICT implementation for persons with dementia in Dementia and first on the international level. May inform regional and national policy makers on caregiver burden Descriptive analysis (univariate and bivariate analyses) Chi square Fisher exact Mann Whitney U t-test ANOVA/ANCOVA Economic analyses (cost of illness, budget impact analysis, cost utility analysis, & probabilistic sensitivity analyses)	The builds on previous promising results of Italian project UP-TECH expected to have a greater impact on caregivers (quality of life and care conditions/ burden)	Relevant study because number of persons living with dementia expected to double from 47.5 million by 2030. Informal caregiving has also increased. Detailed primary and secondary outcomes for persons with dementia and caregivers noted.	Trial status per this article was in recruitment. Final results were unavailable. The initial study did fit search criteria for research inclusive of caregivers and the collection of precision health data.	Studies such as the TECH@home study and similar have the potential to inform policy and affect cost burden and caregiver burden for diseases such as Alzheimer. The collection & integration of health care data collected from wearables and sensors continues to be promising in affecting health for patients and caregivers.	The data provided by technology-infused smart homes can affect the quality of life for both patients and caregivers. Studies may inform policy such as privacy and security concerns. Technology in the home has potential for benefits realized by reducing caregiver burden and burnout as well.
19	Michaud and Turgeon,[7] 2021	Describe the concept of precision medicine and its implementation	Literature review	Not specified	Literature review of 6 articles illustrating pharmacogenomics testing and clinical application of precision medicine	Several clinical and genetic markers were highlighted in the literature review. There were limitations and notable impact for many of the studies.	Precision medicine was promising in the treatment of fibromyalgia based on biomarkers. MiRNomes by MiRNomes by aiding in diagnosis. Precision medicine improved predictive dosing by screening for	The study mentioned several experimental studies although specific details were not listed for many of the studies.	No study-specific details such as reliability coefficients or specific instruments were listed for each study.	The investigators maintain a positive perspective on the multiple uses for pharmacogenomics and precision medicine. The study results shared provide support for implementation and value across several areas of practice and clinical treatment.	Integration of precision medicine is promising across several clinical treatment areas and patient population. Benefits may be realized in several disease processes from diagnosis to treatment. Health care providers are encouraged to investigate its efficacy when determining which drugs should be prescribed and/or treatment programs implemented.

(continued on next page)

Table 1 (continued)

No.	Author/s Date	Research Question	Design & Method	Population Sample (Size, Type)	Data Collection/ Instruments	Analysis	Findings	Strengths	Limitations	Conclusion	Implications (Take Home Message)
						Overall, there is promise in using precision medicine with pharmacogenomic study.	dihydropyrimidine dehydrogenase deficiency (DPD) in metabolism of 5-flourouracil (5-FU). Stem cell transplants and gene variants affecting oral clearance resulting in higher or lower plasma concentrations demonstrated significance. Genetic polymorphisms in CYP450 enzyme may also affect metabolism or profile of drugs intended for the treatment of chronic low back pain. The studies reported positive results in the fields of pediatric transplant care as well as antitumor necrosis factor drugs for pediatric inflammatory bowel disease.				
20	Morandi et al,[15] 2013	Describe the prevalence of potentially inappropriate medications (PIM) in critically ill adults during hospitalization and discharge.	Prospective cohort study	120 individuals aged 60 y and older who survived an ICU hospitalization	APACHE II evaluation, CAM-ICU, Charlson Comorbidity Index BEERS	Poisson regression	250 PIM were prescribed at discharge (opioids, anticholinergics, antidepressants, and orthostatic drugs); 90 of these (36%) were considered actually inappropriate medications (AIM)	Experimental study with sample that would well inform the study due to convenience sampling. Evaluated the clinical situations for prescribing certain medications as clinically feasible.	No mention of multisite or geographic sampling (single center nature) for generalizability. Short- and long-term adverse clinical outcomes and rehospitalization status were also indicated as a limitation. Only prescribed medications, not the cohort was examined. Study was performed before the 2012	Polypharmacy in elderly patients is increasing. Polypharmacy and inappropriate medication prescription is primary cause of adverse events in elderly yet the practice continues.	Potentially inappropriate medications are often prescribed at discharge and often initiated during the ICU stay. The PIMs are often the source of adverse events in the elderly population and warrant an accurate assessment and screening for medical necessity, especially medications with highest risk for adverse events.

#	Author, year	Research question	Type	Population	Design	Summary	Findings	Methods	Limitations	Implications	Notes	Conclusions
21	Prosperi et al,[28] 2018	What are the technical & societal hurdles in precision health?	Literature review	Not specified	Literature review	Several hurdles exist with differentiation between precision health and precision medicine across all phases of model development and deployment. Data sources, study designs, prediction modeling, and translational relevance are areas where hurdles and challenges are prevalent.	Investigators found that researchers focused too much on genetics and/or -omics. Poorly defined target units such as ethnic groups, geographic areas, and social groups were additional hurdles. Types of data sources, measurement issues, and study designs were problematic and riddled with multiple issues. Reliability (reproducibility, replicability, and generalizability) was a challenge as well. Ethical use and reliance on algorithms was also noted.	The investigators used multiple studies covering different facets of precision health challenges. They shared various models and supporting graphics for ease of understanding. The investigators also indicated the potential for bias when using large amounts of data not proportioned to observational or prospective studies.	Limited information available on specific types of studies, reliability measures and methods, and demographics was provided.	Precision health access points such as the EHR and avatar can assist researchers to reach larger populations and create study designs that succeed in examination of rare adverse drug effects where insufficiently powered RCTs cannot. Prediction models are still inaccurate.	BEERS was published with updated criteria; agreement between clinicians was not assessed, resulting in potential bias between panel members.	Public health models must be translatable, reliable, and generalizable. Of importance is the impact of empowerment, which, per the investigators, has the ability to modify behaviors and reduce disease risk in arthritis. Education and integration of policymaking and ethics is paramount to the success of the precision medicine program. The investigators conclude with a requirement for "interdisciplinary expertise and multiple disciplines" and suggests transdisciplinarity, a move beyond disciplines.
22	Shen et al,[8] 2020	How can precision health be used to manage the older patient with cancer?	Online Book Chapter Literature review	Not specified	Literature review	Summary	Several recent studies examined the usefulness of precision medicine and pharmacogenomic testing as well as managing polypharmacy in older adults.	Referenced article is specific to polypharmacy in the older adult and uses precision medicine to improve drug regimens to mitigate polypharmacy and improve safety. The articles list	The selected chapter provided limited information on the specified and highlighted study, requiring additional searches for more detailed information.	Oncologic treatment is but one of the areas showing promise in utilization of health care informatics and technology. Informatics and technology are collection components for the data available from wearables, screening, and data repositories. The continued development of these programs can help direct usage of pharmacologic data from clinical and genetic sources for use in the elderly population.		Smart home technology and wearables are a potential source for data needed to implement precision medicine, which stems from ease of collection and use. Patients may report symptoms, and care can be provided or prescribed real-time according to findings. Translation of the interventions from oncology to other fields of study is imminent.

(continued on next page)

Table 1 (continued)

No.	Author/s Date	Research Question	Design & Method	Population Sample (Size, Type)	Data Collection/ Instruments	Analysis	Findings	Strengths	Limitations	Conclusion	Implications (Take Home Message)
								additional indications and examples for other interventions using precision medicine for comparison.			
23	Sjoding et al,[11] 2016	What are longitudinal changes in ICU admissions among elderly patients?	Retrospective cohort study	27.8 million patients in US Hospitals from 1996 to 2010	Aggregated data from primary ICD-9 codes	SAS 9.2 and STATA 13 were used for analysis. In addition, sensitivity analyses were conducted. ICU case mix was used to graphically represent data. Researchers reviewed fee for service and paid Medicare beneficiaries as well as Medicare beneficiaries with a coronary care or ICU care or ICU room and board charge	Found significant declines in cardiovascular admissions from 26.6% to 12.6% and congestive heart failure from 8.5% to 5.4%. Sepsis admissions, however, increased from 11th rank to 1st rank.	Large sample size, longitudinal study	Specifications were listed for demographics such as age, gender, or geographic location for descriptive data in this report via supplemental link.	Primary diagnoses of critical care patients have changed over a 15-year period. Changes in admissions diagnoses and their prevalence should be monitored for such changes with data collection.	Data show that the elderly is the fastest growing group of patients being admitted to the critical care units. This places them at risk of polypharmacy and make them prime candidates for precision medicine initiatives and research endeavors. Researchers must continue to monitor prevalence of specific diseases over time, as they are highly subject to change.
24	Takahashi et al,[14] 2012	Does telemonitoring in older adults prevent hospitalizations and emergency department visits?	RCT	205 participants	Elder Risk Assessment Index (ERA) Kokmen Short Test of Mental Status Intel Health Guide Charleston Index	Primary outcome was composite endpoint of hospitalizations and emergency department visits in 12 mo following enrollment. Secondary endpoints included hospitalizations, ED visits, and total hospital days; intent-to-treat analysis was performed.	Primary outcome of hospitalizations and ED visits did not differ between the telemonitoring and usual care (57.3%) groups $P = .035$. There were no differences in secondary endpoints and no significant differences between enrollment and preenrollment.	The design of RCT was a strength, as RCTs are a gold standard for experimental studies. The study was multisite and included a rural site.	It was not practical to blind the providers or the patients who received home equipment monitoring due to possible Hawthorne effect and potential bias and improved effect in the interventional group. Some participants outside of the Mayo clinic may not have been recorded. Other demographic factors may have added to differentiation (ie, education, socioeconomic status, transportation, or caregiver or social support). Access to tertiary hospital and case management could have also introduced bias	Researchers proposed that telemonitoring could be the answer to improving outcomes. The study consisted of adults aged 60 y and older. The study, however, did not indicate any significant differences in hospitalization or secondary endpoints. The study group had a mean average of 80.3 y. There was a significant difference in mortality which was higher in the telemonitoring group. The significance in mortality is an implication for future research as its causality is unknown.	The fact that there was no difference in the usual care and intervention group may have reflected the large number of participants. The quality of the monitoring of the intervention group may also be assessed to determine if the platform and telemonitoring was sufficient. Overlap may have been present in the usual care guidelines as compared with the intervention group. Usual care may be sound treatment. Usual care is designed to reduce readmissions and address issues that could prompt hospitalizations. Efforts to improve access to care for elderly with lack

#	Author, Year	Question	Study type	Sample	Instruments	Statistical methods	Findings		Interpretation	Conclusions
							periods. Mortality was higher in the telemonitoring group (14.7%) vs the usual care group (3.9%). The figure was statistically significant (P = .008)	into results and therefore affect generalizability.		of transportation and caregivers are critical to success.
									The study introduces the potential connection to genetic disease and effects of the disease in comparison to the premorbid state. This point reinforces the need for genetic study and/or mapping.	
25	Tasker,[18] 2012	What is the real target of glycemic control and hypoglycemia in pediatric critical care patients?	Literature review (1 RCT, 2-center RCT, 2 retrospective studies)	700 critically ill pediatric patients 456 children (follow-up) 980 children	Not specified	Wilcoxon rank sum tests, 2-sample t-tests, chi square analysis, Kaplan–Meier time-to-vent-analysis. All analyses were done using SAS version 9.1 and performed in blinded manner.	Methods not specified	Tight glycemic control did not change early infection rate, mortality, length of stay, or measures of organ failure. Critically ill children experienced a 15-point decrease in intelligence quotient scores.	Multiple RCTs selected for the review as well as a 2-center RCT, follow-up study conducted on patients of original study	The 2 pediatric tight glycemic control studies were from 2 different time periods (subject to different treatment programs: ie, sepsis guidelines), therefore affecting generalizability.
										There exist multiple parameters for determining the effect of hypoglycemia. The arterial blood gas and glucose value of <40 are but a few measures. Acceptable glucose ranges may provide additional information on normoglycemic goals. The study illustrates that multiple factors could be responsible for the neurocognitive changes aside from hypoglycemia such as the critical illness itself.
26	Taylor and Barcelona de Mendoza,[16] 2017	What is the role of nurse scientists in -omics-based research especially in minority communities?	Literature review	Multiple studies presented without details regarding population sizes	Review summary Instruments not specified	Not specified	Genetic research presents an opportunity for nurse scientists. Despite growth in the -omics research, minority nurse researchers are still lacking especially in genetics; 13% of nursing faculty identity as African American, Latino, or other underrepresented groups. More studies are needed that include both minority,	The study is applicable and of interest to the nurse researcher and provides several studies for the audience's review of historical nursing contributions and national recognition. More importantly, the investigators reiterate the importance of not conducting research for research's sake, but to effect change in environments,	Several of the studies were older than 10 y but are considered seminal works. Funding awards have been primarily awarded to physicians, epidemiologists, and basic or bench scientists. Studies highlighting more recent clinical research findings are lacking.	Nurses can assume roles other than recruitment and may serve successfully as consultants and pPrincipal investigators. Nursing has made significant contributions to genetic research, yet still has not been included on many "interdisciplinary" studies.
										Nurses should take advantage of -omics- and genetic-based education and training. They must continue the work of conducting research on vulnerable populations in an ethical manner, seeking to affect the minority communities as lead scientists. Nurses should also continue to position themselves as members of true interdisciplinary research teams as active members and leaders of research teams.

(continued on next page)

Table 1 (continued)

Author/s No. Date	Research Question	Design & Method	Population Sample (Size, Type)	Data Collection/ Instruments	Analysis	Findings	Strengths	Limitations	Conclusion	Implications (Take Home Message)
						patient populations, and on disease treatment based on findings.				
27 Tebani et al,[29] 2016	Describe the paradigm shift in inborn errors of metabolism in -omics-based strategies in precision medicine.	Integrative literature review (experimental studies)	989 neonatal urine samples (multisite study)	Summary	The current method of diagnosing inborn errors of metabolism is slow. -Omics-based research can produce a faster treatment based action or treatment based collected such as databases and biomarkers. Researchers can search for clinically useful tools rather than conducting research for research's sake.	Informatics and inborn errors of metabolism are new tools to enhance clinical decision-making. Researchers can find a suitable action or diagnosis using bioinformatics.	Multistudy and multisite review providing overview of various projects in which -omics and genome approached have resulted in better disease diagnosis, prevention, and management. Investigators thoroughly detail all types of -omics-based methods.	Genome sequencing can result in high cost and low throughput. An additional limitation is time-consuming library preparation of sequences. Short DNA fragments were also used with amplification. Clinical validity is also a challenge. Finally, multiple steps add potential errors to the workflow and make it complex.	The investigators believe that current medical practice has been disrupted and that precision medicine is affecting the future of medicine. Integrity and quality of sample sizes call for biobanking resources.	The investigators also call for a workforce trained in big data or biomedical information management. The call for education in precision medicine has been repeatedly placed.
28 Waltz et al,[30] 2017	What is team-based care?	Literature review	Not specified	TeamSTEPPS Teamwork Attitude Questionnaire (T-TAQ) TeamSTEPPS Teamwork Perception Questionnaire (T-TPQ) Patient-Reported Outcomes Measurement Information System (PROMIS)	Summary	Team-based care is the method or procedure used to accomplish interprofessional collaborative practice. The investigators reinforce graduate nurses' position as future leaders in education, practice, and research and further underscore other programs' interprofessional aims as part of their accreditation process.	Multiple experimental studies were used, and instruments and tools were valid and reliable. The investigators also state that interprofessional collaborative practice is when different health care professionals work with families, caregivers, patients, and the community	26 instruments measuring teamwork attitudes or perceptions were vetted; however all were not listed.	The interprofessional collaborative practice is called for in the discipline of nursing and in medical curricula as part of accreditation requirements. Unfortunately, nursing is still underrepresented and supporters such as the Josiah Macy foundation provide funding opportunities.	The purpose of nursing-led interprofessional collaborative research must improve access, cost, and quality. The overarching goal of safety should be at the forefront of nursing research.
27						participants and nurse scientists.				

				Databases, summary	Summary of presented studies	Some studies	Multiple	Protein and messenger RNA	Gene expression in children, especially
29	Zimmerman,[19] 2023	What are classic critical care encounters with precision medicine?	Multicenter observational, experimental, observational studies	496 children with shock	Databases, summary Pediatric Risk of Mortality Score, Pediatric SEpsis biomarker Risk modEl (PERSEVERE, PERSEVERE II) Gene Expression Dynamics Inspector	Summary of presented studies	Some studies reported no benefit or harm for the corticosteroid prescription in sepsis. Others showed there was differences in response to certain medications based on differences in genotype.	to achieve optimal health care. Multiple experimental studies used. Investigators reported reliability and confidence intervals as well as statistical significance. Multiple sites were used although all sites were not detailed with regard to geographic location.	Protein and messenger RNA quantification tools are needed to quantify and make clinical decisions. The processes of creating some of the tools is time-consuming and labor-intensive.	Gene expression in children, especially with regard to endotype subclass, genotype, and phenotype, should be considered in clinical decision-making and prescribing. These considerations are important because clinical response differs based on genetic makeup and illness severity. Successful research programs must do more than identify the genes causing disease. They must work to minimize the impact with consideration for the environment and with translation to the clinical environment.

Abbreviations: CCN, critical care nurse; ED, emergency department; RCT, randomized controlled trial; VHA, Veterans Health Administration.

SELECTION PROCESS

An initial computer-assisted search of the keyword "precision medicine" returned more than 3,09,962 sources across 4 databases (OVID, PubMED, Scopus, and Cochrane). Based on readings, redefining the term to "precision health" resulted in 169 sources (**Fig. 1**; PRISMA Diagram). Once potential studies were identified using search strategies, a high-level initial review of these articles and/or their abstracts sought references to assessment scales, caregivers, seniors, critical care, or interprofessional. Several search results after combining terms precision health or precision medicine with "and" or "or" caregiver and polypharmacy returned no results. Alternately, when combining the term "precision health" to "interprofessional" caregivers, 7 results were returned. A keyword combination of the terms precision health and elderly returned 25 results. There were no results incorporating precision

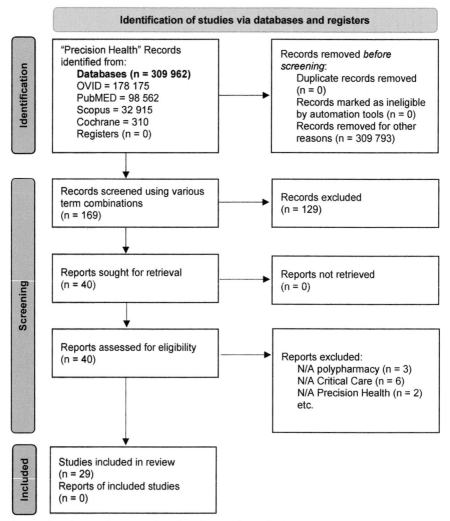

Fig. 1. The PRISMA diagram identifies the number of selected studies and refinement of search strategies. (Created with BioRender.com.)

health, polypharmacy, elderly, critical care, and caregivers. The combination of "precision medicine and "caregiver" returned no results indicating a paucity in the literature.

Thirty-nine articles were iteratively reviewed for inclusion and exclusion criteria based on the topic of interest. Articles that were inclusive of the keywords precision medicine or precision health and critical care met inclusion criteria and were retained. Articles containing precision health and polypharmacy were also retained. Any methodology used was permissible. Articles were excluded if they did not include association to polypharmacy, elderly critical care patients, or caregivers or if they focused on precision health as a determinant of any other model other than assessment of polypharmacy or caregivers of elderly critical care patients. Any unpublished works were also excluded.[18] After multiple iterative reviews and deselecting nonrelated terms, the final results were reviewed for sample size, design, level of evidence, and strong analyses and totaled 29 articles (see **Fig. 1**).

FINDINGS
Precision Health and Technology Usage in the Elderly

Precision health relies on technology to collect, analyze, and store data collected. Within the literature search were beneficial, technological tools for assessment, reporting and tracking of metrics that can provide assistance to both caregivers and health care providers with respect to symptom science.[5,7,10] Through the accurate collection, organization, storage, and reporting of data, genetic and environmental trends can be studied and addressed. Technology has a critical place in our current health care system. Technology such as continuous glucose monitors, smart watches, wellness trackers, and Bluetooth devices can collect results that may correlate to discrepancies in medication adherence, missed doses, or based on symptoms that can provide data for precision health. In the absence of this technology, there is an inherent reliance on the informal caregiver. As such, increased attention should be placed on both the patient and the designated caregiver as an equal partner in polypharmacy risk reduction and help trigger deprescribing of duplicate medications and overlapping therapies. Primary information should be routinely transferred directly from provider to patient/caregiver, thus placing a greater emphasis on opportunities to engage and empower the informal caregiver or family member. By strengthening their role as an advocate with home medication usage and symptom monitor, previously missed assessment data may be shared with the health care team.

NURSING

Nursing has been historically underrepresented in the conduct of research using Big Data or repositories. They are a valued part of the inpatient care team and therefore should also be integral members of the research team.[16] Nursing professionals have unique skillsets in ethics, care planning, safety, quality improvement, and assessment. Nurses also spend considerably more minutes at the bedside with the patients during their shifts compared with medicine or pharmacy at admit, during the hospitalization, and at discharge. Nurses are essential in collection of data and monitoring outcomes of medical treatment (**Fig. 2**). Schools of nursing are beginning to incorporate genetic and pharmacogenomic content into curriculum in an effort to educate nurses on the unique polymorphisms and competition for chemical receptor sites and the way they vary from patient to patient.[31] Nurses may benefit from the study of omics, a targeted approach to understand diseases and the individual patient

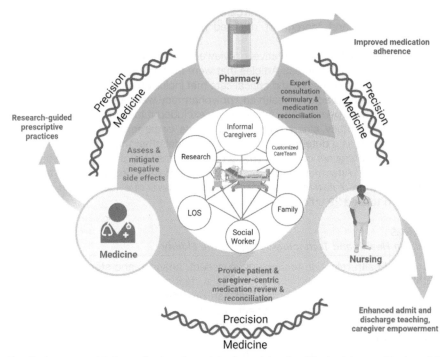

Fig. 2. A proposed interprofessional model of precision health depicts a patient-centric interprofessional approach to pharmacotherapy. The model further illustrates the integration of research using precision medicine by the 3 major disciplines (Medicine, Pharmacy, and Nursing) and the potential areas of impact. (*Adapted from* "Systems Biology Cycle Template", by BioRender.com (2023). Retrieved from https://app.biorender.com/biorender-templates.)

Table 2 Focus areas for nursing knowledge in –omics[a,b,c,d]	
Area	**Definition**
Epigenomics	Study of how the environment affects gene expression
Genomics	Study of all gene interrelationships
Lipidomics	Study of how lipids affect gene expression
Metabolomics	Study of how metabolites affect gene expression
Pharmacodynamics	Study of drugs and their mechanism of action
Pharmacogenetics	Study of the effect of genetic biomarkers on drug response
Pharmacogenomics	Study of the influence of variability of multiple genes on drug response
Pharmacokinetics	Study of drug absorption, distribution, metabolism, and excretion
Proteomics	Study of how proteins affect gene expression

The table provides a list of terms related to the study of –omics. Nurses may focus on these areas of study to enhance their knowledge of –omics. These terms are frequently found throughout published research on precision medicine. Omics: defined as "the study of".

[a] Content adapted from the following sources: Hickey, et al., 2019.
[b] Hull, 2018.
[c] Kurnat-Thoma, Graves & Billones., 2022.
[d] Taylor & Barcelona de Mendoza, 2018.

response to those diseases on a molecular level. Nurses accomplish the tactic through the use of several omics such as genomics, proteomics, metabolomics, and/or pharmacogenomics. **Table 2** defines focus areas for nursing knowledge in pharmacogenomics. A renewed focus on SDoH and geomapping is also in order, as where an individual works, plays, and lives is paramount to managing their chronic diseases. Incorporating precision health, genetic sequencing, informatics, and big data into the nursing curriculum prepares novice nurses to move the nursing profession forward in tandem with emerging scientific innovation.[31] The American Academy of Nursing delivered a national call to increase the number of nurses involved in research and utilization of precision health and nurse leaders, and scientists are tasked with ensuring the profession rises to the that call.[31]

PHARMACY

Pharmacy is perhaps the most evolved in the utilization of precision health, especially pharmacogenomics. Research-driven best practices ensure pharmacists are often noted as consultation experts for off-label usage and genetic-focused prescriptive nuances.[29] For example, pharmacogenomics allow pharmacists to evaluate and prescribe medications that are uniquely targeted to a patient's genetic makeup. Another such example is a drug's mechanism of action and affinity for cellular biomarkers. Based on drug responses, medical professionals can select specific chemotherapy agents or antibiotics and better metabolized drugs.[32] By incorporating data such as metabolism, absorption, and elimination, pharmacodynamic response may affect antibiotic stewardship or eliminate the need to "try out" or "test" medications that can be prescribed based on their genetic complement and pharmacogenes.[32] Possessing extensive backgrounds in Chemistry and biological study of reactions at the cellular and enzymal level, pharmacists are aware of several incompatibilities that may surface when using one drug versus the other and how they vary from population to population. Pharmacists are well versed in implementation of several clinical decision tools such as the Beers Criteria, PRISCUS list, Screening Tool to Alert to Right Treatment (START), Screening Tool of Older Person's Prescriptions (STOPP), and the Drug Burden Index (DBI).[25] Sixty-four percent of the tools use dosing as criteria, whereas 2.4% including the latter tool consider the more specific actual dose used.[9] Pharmacists play a key part in advancing precision medicine initiatives into interprofessional patient care (see **Fig. 2**).

MEDICINE

Physicians are the first to prescribe, augment, or change the medication regimen. Following research-driven treatment guidelines for multiple disease processes, physicians often are at the core of managing the initial prescription, monitoring, and alleviation of symptoms of adverse drug results. Physicians can discover patterns and trends in prescribing and commit to a patient-centric rather than protocol-driven prescribing practice. By connecting with and closely listening to patients, adherence may be improved (see **Fig. 2**). Physicians who take initiative and actively seek to resolve issues and requests without being dismissive of patients or caregivers demonstrate mastery of soft skills of patient care. Balancing the issues of access, affordability, and adherence is a delicate act in today's health care climate. Although economic reasons may prevent patients from adhering to the prescribed regimen, less attention is often given to the genetic polymorphisms that cause one person to react to a medication differently than another. Polymorphisms may act on multiple drug pathways. In the setting of polypharmacy, there are multiple drugs acting on numerous pathways for compounded effect and clearance. Two examples of polymorphisms at play are interactions between drugs and the CYP2D6 and CYP2C19.[25] Clearance and interaction between metoprolol and citalopram and citalopram and omeprazole, respectively, are affected by clearance.[25] A tailored drug prescription, treatment, and monitoring is the very essence of precision medicine.[1,7,9,10,23,25,32] Clinical research may add to the notion that drugs are not broadly created and prescribed among general populations but rather tailored to an individual person based on their genetic makeup.[23] Optimal response to therapy is the goal of genetic-directed therapies.

INTERPROFESSIONAL APPROACH

The interprofessional approach focuses on communication and a mutual understanding of and respect for each team member's role and/or contribution to patient care. Likewise, the patient is also considered a member of the team. Therefore, in the absence of a cognitively intact patient, the family member or informal caregiver steps into that role. The literature also indicates patients/caregivers should share an equal partnership with researchers engaged in research using their patient's precision health data.[20] In order to mitigate negative outcomes associated with polypharmacy in elderly critical care patients, nurses must be educated in matters of precision health, especially pharmacogenomics (see **Table 2**). The final checkpoint in the drug administration pathway are nurses armed with expertise in assessment based on pharmacogenetic nuances, resulting in increased patient safety. An example of one such nuance is when a patient's endotype (genetic subclass) affects their response to corticosteroids in sepsis.[19] Two patients with different endotypes can have very different reactions to medications. Using a communication tool such as SBAR, which represents situation, background, assessment, and recommendations, *recommendations* can be made based on best practices in medication administration and patient teaching. Nursing is key to fostering interprofessional and truly collaborative team practice.

The Institute of Medicine's *Future of Nursing* report indicates research, education, and practice as areas designated in which future nurse graduates and leaders may emerge.[30] A heightened focus can then be placed on family and caregiver teaching, empowering them to speak up concerning challenges with their medication regimen and accurate reporting of untoward effects. When the entire interprofessional team truly places the patient and caregiver dyad at the center of care, a 2-way stream of open communication occurs and facilitates a move toward safety in medication administration. As nurses often monitor their patient's postadministration of regularly prescribed and investigative medications for clinical trials, a deeper understanding of the pharmacodynamics and pharmacokinetics can encourage their growth as nurse scientists and increase their involvement in research.

The informal caregiver who is involved and engaged in the plan of care understands the indications for prescribed medications. Often at the bedside during hospitalization, the informal caregiver is witness to manifestations of drug side effects and whether the intended affect is achieved with the exception of vital signs and other clinical parameters. Most inappropriate medications prescribed are first initiated in the ICU.[15] According to a study by Morandi and others, 100% of muscle relaxants, 71% of atypical anticholinergics, and 67% of nonbenzodiazepines and benzodiazepines were classified as actually inappropriate medications.[15] When determining which medications should be continued on discharge, the feedback of the physician, pharmacist, nursing staff, and the caregiver or family should be considered to determine which medications are truly clinically necessary. In addition, empowering the informal caregiver or family member by soliciting their input may encourage the same when visiting other specialty providers to have the conversation about potential drug interactions before introducing new medications or resuming others.

SYNTHESIS OF LITERATURE
Discussion

On reviewing the state of science regarding precision health as a model for assessment of caregiver impact on polypharmacy of elderly patients hospitalized in ICUs, this researcher determined a need for an interprofessional precision health model for caregivers of elderly ICU patients due to the lack of research studies on the subject. Findings from the literature review of randomized controlled trials and observational studies presented opportunities for future research, incorporating precision health and caregivers with a focus on elderly patients in critical care units. Opportunities are abundant for interprofessional precision health studies involving medicine, nursing, and polypharmacy due to the lack of studies in which nursing is adequately represented. The limited number of nurse-led research studies involving interprofessional use of precision health shows that more work is needed to foster interprofessional research and implement a team-based approach to health care using precision health. Only 11 of the articles mentioned collaboration with nursing using precision medicine or omics.[2,3,5,10,16,20,25,29–34] Calling for interprofessional or interdisciplinary research, as did several of the investigators in their works, does not reflect what is currently occurring in practice.[2,4,10,16,24,30] Limiting or omitting the role of the nurse in major genetic studies is commonplace and counterproductive. The roles of nurse researchers should warrant professional respect.[32] The nurse researcher should also have an integral role in the research team in leadership or as a principal or coinvestigator and not relegated to the menial tasks of data collection.[4,16] Nurses bring a different perspective and wealth of expertise. The interprofessional nature of the team may even be expanded to include social workers and respiratory therapists as well as the community health care worker.[30] The 4 articles that touted engaging the informal caregiver again indicate a paucity in the literature and an opportunity for more in-depth research.[3,12,24,26]

IMPLICATIONS FOR PRACTICE, POLICY, RESEARCH, AND EDUCATION

Nursing practice is constantly evolving in conjunction with health care. Nurses with educational backgrounds in –omics are able to assess, examine, analyze, and propose tailored treatments by incorporating aggregated precision health data. Graduate nurses are better prepared to navigate complex patient care due to multiple comorbidities and polypharmacy with foundational knowledge of genetic indicators and symptom expressions. It is highly recommended to add the term and related terminology, for precision health to the scope and standards of practice for entry-level and advanced nurses. This addition will serve as a constant guide to approach nursing practice through a lens of customized and personalized care. Nursing theory is based on multiple concepts and frameworks. Several theories suggest the provision of holistic care that is inclusive of the whole patient, which always includes the patient, family, and/or caregiver (formal or informal). Additional research is needed on the influence or impact of the informal caregiver on patient outcomes.

Advocacy for communities burdened with inequity in health care access, housing, food insecurity, and high prescription costs for nonformulary drugs has always been and should continue to be a nurse-led initiative. These economic influences shape the manner patients manage their medication regimens, often with most factors out of their control. Prevalent precision health findings encountered in daily nursing practice may spur calls for legislative lobbying action and policy formation. One such example is lowering the cost of prescription medications. Data from precision health efforts may indicate geographic areas of concern that suggest target areas for research funding and support to improve patient outcomes. Nurses competent in precision health, as it pertains to polypharmacy, assert that access to genetically ideal medication is more than an SDoH, but in fact, a political one that varies across communities, economic strata, and zip codes.[32,35]

Research and education are intricately intertwined. The continued call for an increased number of nursing scientists matches the demands of an evolving health care landscape in which practitioners are both research scholars and providers. There exists a need for research targeting nursing knowledge (research-focused) and patient-focused clinical practice (research by advanced practice nurses), thus translating research to the clinical bedside. Nurses must first be educated and competent in advanced concepts such as precision health and –omics-based health care.[25,29,31–33] Once nurses understand the methods in which precision health can benefit critically ill elderly patients and minimize the risks of polypharmacy, they can truly embrace their research potential to affect outcomes.[31] Organizations such as NIH and the NINR encourage the development of future nurse researchers through the provision of fellowships, educational offerings, and funding announcements earmarked to entice and professionally develop the burgeoning researcher.[3] The lack of research studies found on this topic indicate an opportunity to add to the nursing body of knowledge.

Educators have the responsibility to lay the foundation of precision health education in schools of nursing. Purposefully weaving the content across the nursing curriculum allows the potential nurse researcher to understand its application across multiple practice areas and health conditions. Academic health care partners with robust medical research departments engaged in clinical drug research can also offer clinical immersion programs for interested nursing students and new nurses. Through structured volunteer or educational opportunities, precision health knowledge is introduced regarding its use as well as the process for clinical and investigative drug research trials.

SUMMARY

Nursing professionals remain underrepresented in research involving precision health. Although there is limited research on nursing, precision health, and the critically ill elder patient, the symptom science branch has shown promise as an area for nurses to conduct relevant and germane research that can improve outcomes. The paucity in the literature illuminates multiple implications for future research. Examples emerged such as interprofessional approaches to polypharmacy, caregiver impact on polypharmacy at various points along the critical illness trajectory, and ethical dilemmas related to precision health in the target population. Strategic initiatives designed to increase the number of nurses involved in transformational research should continue to be funded as well as programs geared to develop novice nurse researchers. Schools of nursing, academic health care facilities, and academic-practice partnerships should continue to receive fiscal support to educate and professionally develop nurse researchers on precision health methods and their impact on health care. As such, all health care is an interprofessional initiative. Research should reflect these interprofessional contributions accordingly with representation from all disciplines engaged in safe pharmaceutical practices.

CLINICS CARE POINTS

- Further research is needed to fully assess caregiver impact on precision health and polypharmacy.
- A reliable and validated assessment tool or instrument should be developed to capture data on caregiver impact on polypharmacy.
- Precision health data should be collected to better direct clinical care, especially prescribing practices.
- Health care providers should hone and use soft skills (ie, connecting with and listening to patients) during interactions with patients to accurately gather responses to medications.
- Precision health and polypharmacy monitoring and initiatives should use an interprofessional and team-based approach to address issues from all relevant perspectives and vantage points.
- Engaging both formal and informal caregivers in addition to family at the bedside during rounds or during huddles is key for accurate history taking, medication review, and reconciliation.
- Do not assume nonadherence without further investigation of patient, family, or informal caregiver feedback.

REFERENCES

1. Collins FS, Varmus H. A new initiative on precision medicine. N Engl J Med 2015; 372(9):793–5.
2. Hickey KT, Bakken S, Byrne MW, et al. Precision health: advancing symptom and self-management science. Nurs Outlook 2019;67(4):462–75.
3. Hull SC. Are we ready for precision health? Nurs Manag 2018;49(7):9–11.
4. Javier S, Zimmerman L, Kimerling R. Measuring Ethnicity and race using the common data model: implications for precision in health disparities research. Health Serv Res 2020;55(S1):45–6.
5. Karolak A, Markov DA, McCawley LJ, et al. Towards personalized computational oncology: from spatial models of tumour spheroids, to organoids, to tissues. J R Soc Interface 2018;15(138):20170703.
6. Majumder S, Emad Aghayi, Noferesti M, et al. Smart homes for elderly health-care—recent advances and research challenges. Sensors 2017;17(11):2496.
7. Michaud V, Turgeon J. Precision medicine: applied concepts of pharmacogenomics in patients with various diseases and polypharmacy. Pharmaceutics 2021;13(197):1–3.
8. Shen J, Xie Z, Naeim A. Healthcare informatics and technology in managing the older cancer patient. Geriatric Oncology 2017;1–12. https://doi.org/10.1007/978-3-319-44870-1_89-1.
9. Cacchione PZ. Precision medicine an interprofessional science. Clin Nurs Res 2016;25(4):359–61.
10. Gameiro G, Sinkunas V, Liguori G, et al. Precision Medicine: changing the way we think about healthcare. Clinics 2018;73. https://doi.org/10.6061/clinics/2017/e723.
11. Sjoding MW, Prescott HC, Wunsch H, et al. Longitudinal changes in ICU admissions among elderly patients in the United States. Crit Care Med 2016;44(7):1353–60.

12. Bossen AL, Kim H, Williams KN, et al. Emerging roles for telemedicine and smart technologies in dementia care. Smart Homecare Technol TeleHealth 2015;3: 49–57.

13. TeamSTEPPS 2.0. www.ahrq.gov. Accessed 2023. https://www.ahrq.gov/teamstepps/instructor/index.html.

14. Takahashi PY, Pecina JL, Upatising B, et al. A randomized controlled trial of tele-monitoring in older adults with multiple health issues to prevent hospitalizations and Emergency department visits. Arch Intern Med 2012;172(10). https://doi.org/10.1001/archinternmed.2012.256.

15. Morandi A, Vasilevskis E, Pandharipande PP, et al. Inappropriate medication prescriptions in elderly adults surviving an intensive care unit hospitalization. J Am Geriatr Soc 2013;61(7):1128–34.

16. Taylor JY, Barcelona de Mendoza V. Improving -Omics-Based research and precision health in minority populations: recommendations for nurse scientists. J Nurs Scholarsh 2017;50(1):11–9.

17. New Chartbook Highlights Current Challenges in Patient Safety. www.ahrq.gov. Published 2023. https://www.ahrq.gov/news/ptsafety-chartbook.html. Accessed May 8, 2023.

18. Tasker RC. Pediatric critical care, glycemic control, and hypoglycemia. JAMA 2012;308(16):1687.

19. Zimmerman JJ. The classic critical care conundrum encounters precision medicine. Pediatr Crit Care Med 2023;24(3):251–3.

20. Kluwe F, Michelet R, Mueller-Schoell A, et al. Perspectives on model-informed precision dosing in the digital health Era: challenges, opportunities, and recommendations. Clinical Pharmacology & Therapeutics 2020;109(1):29–36.

21. Alishahi Sevick C, Mathieu S, Everhart R, et al. No-show rates for telemedicine versus in-person appointments during the COVID-19 pandemic: implications for medicaid populations. J Ambul Care Manag 2022;45(4):332–40.

22. Akroute AR, Bondas T. Critical care nurses and relatives of elderly patients in intensive care unit–Ambivalent interaction. Intensive Crit Care Nurs 2016; 34(34):67–80.

23. Ashley EA. The precision medicine initiative. JAMA 2015;313(21):2119.

24. Chi NC, Demiris G. A systematic review of telehealth tools and interventions to support family caregivers. J Telemed Telecare 2014;21(1):37–44.

25. Fujita K, Masnoon N, Mach J, et al. Polypharmacy and precision medicine. Cambridge Prisms: Precision Medicine 2023;1:1–32.

26. Malmgren Fänge A, Schmidt SM, Nilsson MH, et al. The TECH@HOME study, a technological intervention to reduce caregiver burden for informal caregivers of people with dementia: study protocol for a randomized controlled trial. Trials 2017;18(1). https://doi.org/10.1186/s13063-017-1796-8.

27. Morgan D, Swetenham K, To T, et al. Telemonitoring via self-report and video review in community palliative care: a case report. Healthcare 2017;5(3):51.

28. Prosperi M, Min JS, Bian J, Modave F. Big data hurdles in precision medicine and precision public health. BMC Med Inform Decis Mak 2018;18(1):139.

29. Tebani A, Afonso C, Marret S, et al. Omics-based strategies in precision medicine: toward a paradigm shift in inborn Errors of metabolism investigations. Int J Mol Sci 2016;17(9). https://doi.org/10.3390/ijms17091555.

30. Waltz C, Strickland O, Lenz E. Measurement in nursing and health research. 5th edition. Philadelphia, PA: Springer Publishing Company; 2017.

31. Fangonil-Gagalang E, Schultz MA. Diffusion of precision health into a baccalaureate nursing curriculum. J Nurs Educ 2021;60(2):107–10.

32. Kessler C. Genomics and precision medicine: implications for critical care. AACN Adv Crit Care 2018;29(1):28–35.
33. Quinn W, O'Brien E, Springan G. AARP public policy Institute, PPI. AARP. 2018. Available at: http://www.aarp.org/ppi/. Accessed May 8, 2023.
34. Khan T, Eschbach C, Cuthbertson CA, et al. Connecting Primary Care to Community-Based Education: Michigan Physicians' Familiarity With Extension Programs. Health Promot Pract 2020;21(2):175–80.
35. Kurnat-Thoma EL, Graves LY, Billones RR. A Concept Development for the Symptom Science Model 2.0. Nurs Res 2022;71(6):E48–60.

Transition of Care for Older Adults Undergoing General Surgery

Elissa Persaud, MSN, RN, ACCNS-AG, CCRN-CSC[a],*,
Courtney Nissley, MS, RN, AGCNS-BC, CMSRN[b],
Eric Piasecki, MSN, RN, APRN, ACCNS-AG, CCRN, TCRN, SCRN[b],
Carrie Quinn, MSN, RN, ACCNS-AG, CPAN, CNL-BC[b]

KEYWORDS

- Preoperative • Geriatric • Handoff • Discharge • Clinical nurse specialist

KEY POINTS

- Older adults undergoing surgery are at high risk for perioperative complications.
- Providing clear handoff communication during transitions of care can reduce the risk of errors.
- The use of standardized order sets, checklists, and communication templates can improve outcomes in critical care.
- Older adults require specialized care in the postoperative period to avoid functional decline.
- The interprofessional team must collaborate during discharge planning for the older adult to prevent readmission and poor outcomes.

INTRODUCTION

Nearly two decades ago, the National Institute of Medicine published two distinct calls to action, highlighting the need for broad-reaching performance improvement in light of the fact that approximately 98,000 lives are lost at the hands of medical errors each year in the United States.[1,2] In each of these documents, researchers and policy-makers highlighted care transitions as especially error-prone. The older adult population present with unique needs and physiologic changes that further complicate transitions of care, as made plain by researchers who recently observed that approximately 1 in 7 older adults are readmitted to the hospital within 30 days of discharge following a surgical procedure.[3] Accordingly, galvanizing resources required to care

[a] Michigan Medicine, 1500 East Medical Center Drive, Ann Arbor, MI 48109-5866, USA; [b] Penn Medicine Lancaster General Hospital, 555 North Duke Street, Lancaster, PA 17602, USA
* Corresponding author.
E-mail address: epersaud@med.umich.edu

Crit Care Nurs Clin N Am 35 (2023) 453–467
https://doi.org/10.1016/j.cnc.2023.05.009
0899-5885/23/Published by Elsevier Inc.
ccnursing.theclinics.com

for a growing population of geriatric patients safely and effectively remains a primary concern for the United States health systems and individual clinicians alike.

In a fee-for-service model, the complexity of managing the functional, emotional, intellectual, and physical ramifications of aging in a coordinated and holistic manner proves challenging, as current reimbursement models drive clinicians and payers to focus granularly on the human condition.[4] Perhaps more complex, periods of care transition prove uniquely error-prone and require skilled communication among multiple stakeholders in order to prevent harm and optimize outcomes across the continuum of care.[5] As advanced practice registered nurses with specialized training in translating evidence into clinical practice and using implementation science methodologies, Clinical Nurse Specialists (CNSs) are well poised to improve care transitions for the older adult population.[6] In particular, Adult-Gerontology Clinical Nurse Specialists provide advanced nursing care, ethical decision-making support, consultation, conduct research, translate and implement best practices, enhance communication around geriatric care issues from the bedside to the board room, and serve as role models as a clinical expert for clinical staff caring for the older adult population.[7,8]

TRANSITION OF CARE FROM OUTPATIENT TO PERIOPERATIVE ENVIRONMENT

Older adults have unique needs and require a different level of care in the perioperative setting, as the risk for postoperative morbidity and mortality is higher than their younger counterparts. The presence of comorbidities, location of surgical site, and urgency of surgery are all factors that increase risk. The perioperative continuum of care begins when the need for a surgical intervention is identified. The settings and circumstances can vary. Planned elective surgical procedures offer enhanced preoperative evaluation and planning ability, whereas emergency surgery does not. The decision to proceed with surgery should account for the older adult's health care goals and treatment preferences, inclusive of advanced directives. Consideration should also be given to the anticipated impact of the surgical intervention on disease management, function, burden of care, living situation, and survival.[9] The CNS supports surgical team members in applying the Institute for Healthcare Improvement's (IHI) 4Ms (**Fig. 1**) of high-quality care for older adults (mobility, medication, mentation, and what matters) in the surgical environment.[9,10]

Preoperative Phase of Care

Confirmation and documentation of patient goals and treatment preferences, including advanced directives, should be completed in the preoperative phase of care. In patients with existing advanced directives, patients and caregivers should understand any new risks associated with surgery, and an approach for any life-saving interventions should be determined as part of the informed consent process. Routine suspension of Do-Not-Resuscitate orders in the operative environment is not recommended.[9] The surgical plan and approach for resuscitative measures should align with the patient's values and preferences and support the patient's right to self-determination.[10]

Preoperatively, patients should be screened for risk factors that increase vulnerability to surgical risk. These risk factors include advanced older age (>85 years), cognitive impairment, delirium, impaired functional status, impaired mobility, malnutrition, and aspiration risk. Older adults undergoing planned elective procedures should have a preoperative fasting period that allows for the intake of clear liquids up to 2 hours before the scheduled procedure, although clinical judgment should be exercised for comorbidities that may increase the risk for aspiration.[11]

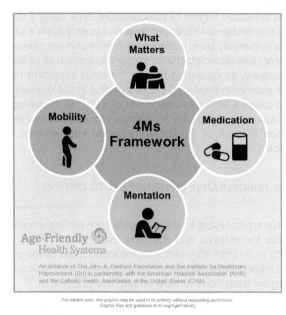

What Matters

Know and align care with each older adult's specific health outcome goals and care preferences including, but not limited to, end-of-life care, and across settings of care.

Medication

If medication is necessary, use Age-Friendly medication that does not interfere with What Matters to the older adult, Mobility, or Mentation across settings of care.

Mentation

Prevent, identify, treat, and manage dementia, depression, and delirium across settings of care.

Mobility

Ensure that older adults move safely every day in order to maintain function and do What Matters.

Fig. 1. Institute for Healthcare Improvement's 4Ms. (*Data from* Institute for Healthcare Improvement. Age-Friendly Health Systems [2023].)

It is standard practice to remove personal belongings and assistive devices (ie, eyeglasses, hearing aids, dentures, and mobility aides) before entering the surgical suite. Prompt return of these items in the immediate postoperative period affects functional recovery of the patient after surgery. Prophylactic antibiotics should be administered preoperatively within 60 minutes before surgical incision. Antibiotic selection should be based on procedure type, risk factors, and the hospital pathogen profile. General surgical procedures, including those in the abdomen, procedures for cancer, bowel anastomosis, and emergent procedures are at higher risk for surgical site infection.[10]

Intraoperative Phase of Care

Intraoperative considerations for the older adult are important, as this population has a decreased reserve to respond to physiologic stress. Key components of intraoperative management include the anesthetic approach, analgesic plan, and postoperative nausea and vomiting prophylaxis.[10]

The older adult population have decreased muscle mass and metabolic rate, predisposing them to perioperative hypothermia and increasing the risk of mortality. Promotion of normothermia during the perioperative continuum is essential to reduce the risk of complications. Maintenance of a core temperature greater than 36° Celsius through the use of patient warming techniques such as forced-warm air or warmed intravenous fluids is used to mitigate risk. Core temperature should be monitored in surgeries lasting longer than 30 minutes.[10]

Risk for Perioperative Pressure Injuries

Accentuated bony prominences, skin condition, decreased muscle tissue and activity, decreased subcutaneous fat, diminished peripheral circulation, and poor nutrition status increase the older adult's risk of developing pressure injuries (PI).[9] All patients, including older adults, should be assessed for risk of perioperative PI by using a validated tool in conjunction with a comprehensive preoperative and postoperative skin assessment. The Braden scale is commonly used in the hospital environment; however, it does not incorporate inherent risks associated with surgery. Common to all validated tools is the duration of surgery, as operating time is the most important risk factor to consider. Every 1-hour extension beyond 6 hours duration in the operating room has been demonstrated to cause a 96% increase in risk of a PI.[12] In the perioperative environment, the CNS supports nursing care workflows, documentation, and preventative strategies to reduce the risk of PI. Evidence-based interventions to reduce risk are highlighted in **Box 1**.

TRANSITION OF CARE FROM THE PERIOPERATIVE ENVIRONMENT TO CRITICAL CARE

Transitions from the perioperative environment to the intensive care setting encompass a wide range of risk points for patients and the care team alike.[13–16] As of more than 2 decades ago, adults older than 65 years encompassed most of the patients undergoing surgery in the United States, further emphasizing the need to understand the complexity of postsurgical transitions of care among this population.[17]

In a recent study on the incidence and prevalence of medical errors in the intensive care setting, researchers categorized 45 out of 120 adverse events among 79 unique patients as preventable.[15] Using failure mode effects analysis, researchers subsequently identified several key points of risk in the transition of patient care from the perioperative to the intensive care environment. Failure modes most common in the perioperative phase of care included failure to (1) provide advanced notification to the critical care team pending case closure, (2) confirm the readiness of the critical care team for patient arrival before initiating transport, (3) communicate the need for a ventilator, (4) have the ventilator ready for patient arrival in the critical care room, and (5) assess the bed and equipment used to transfer the patient from the perioperative setting to the critical care environment.[15] Failures identified in the critical care environment during the transition from the perioperative environment included failure of (1) key team members being present at bedside during the verbal handoff of vital clinical information, (2) record accurate surgical drain output in the immediate postoperative period, (3) place accurate postoperative care orders in a timely fashion.[16]

Box 1
Interventions that may reduce the risk of perioperative pressure injuries

- Using preoperative and postoperative positioning that is different from the intended surgical position
- Providing pressure redistributing support surfaces and padding
- Elevating the heels off the bed, with slight knee flexion, and supporting the calves without pressure on the Achilles tendon or popliteal vein
- Applying prophylactic dressing to protect bony prominences
- Repositioning when possible; may not entail full body movement (eg, micro turn, micro shift)
- Using pressure mapping to provide visual cues to guide repositioning

Data from Association of periOperative Registered Nurses (2022). Interventions to Reduce Pressure Injury.

Seeking to address prior identified gaps in care transition, numerous studies demonstrate the benefit of structured handoff frameworks. Many handoff frameworks include the use of cognitive aides such as checklists to enhance communication of critical patient information among the sending and receiving care teams.[18–22] In addition, standardized education around handoff structure and communication may improve patient safety during transitions from the intraoperative phase of care to the critical care environment.[18,20] Clinicians may consider the implementation of frameworks such as the I-PASS Handoff Communication Template (**Table 1**) or HATRICC (handoffs and transition in critical care) mnemonics when evaluating the potential to guide handoff process improvement.[23] Clinical teams seeking to decrease the risk for error in the perioperative to critical care handoff should also consider communication to the receiving team upstream of the patient's physical transition to critical care as early as 90 minutes before patient transport.[16]

In addition to observing a standard process for perioperative to critical care unit handoff, institutions may benefit from including clinicians such as gerontologists and adult-gerontology–certified advanced practice nurses in handoff and posthandoff evaluation of the older adult.[24–26] Providing advanced nursing care for geriatric patients, adult-gerontology CNSs integrate care of the geriatric patient across the continuum. Whereas other providers focus on the medical management and procedural aspects of transitional care to the critical care environment, the CNS possesses advanced specialty knowledge, population-specific training, translation of evidence into practice, critical thinking regarding the nursing plan of care, and clinical inquiry to identify process and care gaps in situ. Furthermore, CNSs leverage vertical and horizontal system integration to trend opportunities for improvement across multiple patient transitions and subsequently lead the interprofessional team to address gaps using current evidence-based strategies.[6]

Table 1		
I-PASS handoff communication template		
I	Illness severity	Initiate the hand-off report by stating the *severity* of the patient's condition (eg, stable, unstable, critical). Provide the patient's name and current location to the recipient.
P	Patient summary	Share the patient *summary*, including health history, vital signs, surgical procedure, allergies, medical history, and other relevant information pertinent to the patient's current condition.
A	Action list	Include information about *actions* needed, such as priority interventions and a timeline for transfer of care. Present assessment findings and observations of the patient's present and chief complaint, vital signs, symptoms, and diagnoses.
S	Situation awareness and contingency plans	Describe the current *situation*, including code status, level of (un)certainly, recent changes, and response to treatment. Discuss the plan for what may happen.
S	Synthesis by receiver	Ensure that the information related was received accurately. *Synthesis* by the receiver closes the loop of communication, ensuring that the information related was received accurately.

Data from Elsevier. Skills: Hand-off Report: Nursing Report – CE. elsevierperformancemanager.com.

Management of the Older Adult in Critical Care

The older adult population is at a high risk of developing complications while in the critical care environment. Complications that arise while a patient is in critical care may lead to functional decline from prolonged ventilation, immobilization, and insufficient nutrition. The CNS could round on high-risk patients daily to track and trend patient progress and intervene as needed. Because the CNS acknowledges the patient as a whole, rather than an admission diagnosis, these advanced practice nurses are skilled in using various resources that can decrease the risk of complications and promote optimal patient outcomes.

The CNS promotes the integration of checklists, guidelines, and protocols into developing order sets to assist with provider and nursing practice workflow.[27,28] Checklists can improve workflow by integrating reminders into daily care to ensure standards are met. Furthermore, incorporating evidence-based care by implementing a comprehensive multicomponent checklist for routine intensive care unit care (**Table 2**) for the older adult population is recommended to achieve optimal outcomes.[24]

There are various resources available to assist in meeting the older adult's needs in the critical care environment. In addition to collaboration with a CNS, consultation with a geriatrician can also be beneficial. A geriatrician's engagement in the health management of the older adult may help the intensivists and hospitalists to focus on acute illness in the critical care and postcritical care management. Shared decision-making through collaboration across disciplines can facilitate safe transitions of care.[24,27] The CNS rounding on high-risk patients allows for vigilance from the clinical expert that helps prevent error.

A serious complication that often affects older adults is delirium. It has been widely proved that the critical care setting may contribute to delirium; therefore, a multidisciplinary approach to delirium management is imperative, as the care for the older adult is complex.[29] Best practice for delirium is prevention through use of multicomponent bundles, as there is currently no Food and Drug Administration–approved delirium treatment.[30] The Society of Critical Care Medicine's Pain, Agitation/Sedation, Delirium, Immobility, and Sleep Disruption (PADIS) guidelines were implemented to reduce iatrogenic risk factors that lead to poor outcomes.[30] The PADIS guidelines recommend dexmedetomidine when a patient is at high risk for delirium or when delirium-associated agitation impedes weaning or extubation from mechanical ventilation.[24,30] In addition, to identify risk factors and facilitate early identification of delirium, the PADIS guidelines recommend utilization of a valid and reliable screening tool, such as the Confusion Assessment Methods for Critical Care (CAM-ICU) or Intensive Care Delirium Screening Checklist (ICDSC) with nonpharmacologic interventions.[24] The CNS drives use of frameworks to affect outcomes.

TRANSITION OF CARE FROM CRITICAL CARE TO THE ACUTE CARE SETTING

Interventions implemented throughout the continuum of care should focus on patient needs and illness management to reduce readmissions and prevent adverse outcomes.[31] The CNS collaborates with providers in the transition of care, helping to allocate appropriate resources that foster improved health management and avoid readmission.[31] Ensuring that the elements of a comprehensive, multicomponent checklist for routine critical care are personalized and integrated into the care plan establishes safeguards for successful transition to the acute care setting.[23]

Communication is a fundamental component that is essential in the care transition process. Older adults are vulnerable to poor handoff due to their acute illnesses,

Table 2
Comprehensive multicomponent checklist for routine intensive care unit (ICU) care

Principle	Routine Practice Suggestion
Prevention of delirium	• Provide patients with hearing aids and glasses • Implement ABCDEF bundle[†] • Minimize use of restraints and tethers
Sleep	• Earplugs, minimization of noise • Conversion to daytime bolus feeds to decrease night-time interruptions[†]
Cognition	• Cognitive stimulation activities such as music, family-voice reorientation, and family involvement
Mood	• Screening for depressive symptoms in patients with prolonged ICU admissions, with referral to psychiatry as needed • Not suggested to screen acutely unwell, newly admitted patients[†]
Mobility and early rehabilitation	• Early physiotherapy or occupational therapy assessment for advancing mobility and function toward maintenance of activities of daily living
Nutrition	• Dietitian consult • Prompt correction of dehydration
Continence	• Removal of indwelling catheters to avoid catheter-associated bladder infections and promote mobility • Maintenance of regular bowel movements
Skin integrity	• Frequent turning to avoid pressure injuries
Minimization of polypharmacy	• Daily medication review by pharmacist using STOPP/START criteria[17] or American Geriatrics Society Beers criteria[18] of potentially inappropriate medications • Monitor new high-risk medications (antipsychotics, sedative-hypnotics, opioids) with a plan to taper or discontinue while in ICU[†]
Environmental modifications to facilitate physical and cognitive function	• Large clocks and calendars • Handrails, uncluttered hallways to allow mobilization • Elevated toilet seats and door levers (not knobs) • Paint colors that emphasize earth tones with contrast between floor, wall, and ceiling, to aid patients with impaired depth perception
Early discharge planning	• Early involvement of social worker and family • Multidisciplinary team rounding with early ongoing emphasis on the goal of returning home (or to prehospital living environment)

Abbreviations: ACE, acute care of the elderly; ICU, intensive care unit; START, screening tool to alert to right treatment; STOPP, screening tool of older person's prescriptions.
Data from Geen, O., Rochwerg, B., & Wang, X.M. Optimizing care for critically ill older adults. Canadian Medical Association Journal. 2021;193(39). doi:10.1503/cmaj.21065.

complex history, and the potential for complications related to decreased monitoring compared with the critical care environment.[32] The plan and goals of care must be documented and communicated to all team members in order to mitigate gaps and duplication of care management.[31] As the patient progresses from the acute stages of illness in the critical care environment, the multidisciplinary team must be mindful of promptly discontinuing medications before the patient's transfer. In addition, critical care orders and nonadherence to standards may hinder the trajectory for a patient in the acute care setting and create long-term complications. These orders may include nothing by mouth, restraints, or bedrest orders.[27]

The CNS plays a key role in identifying challenges for the nurses, patients, and organization while assisting in alleviating barriers through the use of evidence-based interventions.[31] For example, components of postintensive care syndrome (PICS) (**Fig. 2**) are challenges that affect the body as a whole, including, but not limited to, the physical, cognitive, and mental health well-being as well as the quality of life of both the patient and family.[24,30] Because the aging adult is more prone to acute medical events due to disease processes, at least one of the PICS impairments affects more than half of the critical care population.[24,30,32] The evidence-based ABCDEF bundle, listed in **Table 2** Comprehensive Multicomponent Checklist for Routine ICU Care, includes practice interventions that the CNS can help to implement in the critical care environment to reduce the development of PICS.[24,30] Although the CNS is skilled

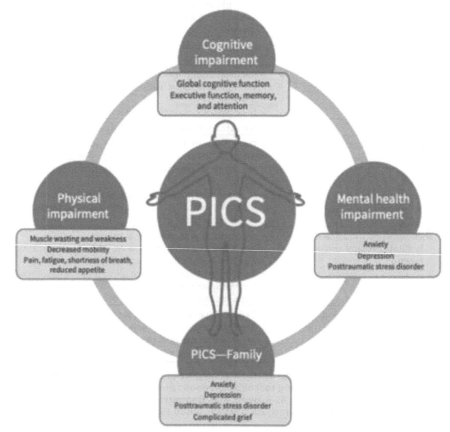

Fig. 2. Components of postintensive care syndrome (PICS). Survivors of the intensive care unit (ICU) may experience cognitive, physical, and mental health impairments. Family members may also experience mental health impairments after the care of a loved one in the ICU. (*Data from* Geen, O., Rochwerg, B., & Wang, X.M. Optimizing care for critically ill older adults. Canadian Medical Association Journal. 2021;193(39). https://doi.org/10.1503/cmaj. 210652.)

at integrating geriatric-focused practices in critical care, it is important to remember that staff engagement is vital in creating sustainable change at the bedside.

Sleep-wake patterns may influence cognitive deficits and development of delirium. Sleep plays a vital role in recovering and healing the mind, body, and spirit.[30] An increase in sleep disruption correlates with functional decline and impaired cognition in the older adult population.[32] The CNS can assist with identifying gaps and developing pathways and bundles for the critical care staff to mitigate the decline. Interventions such as consultation with a dietician for assessment of nutritional status and physical and occupational therapy to assist with early mobilization have been proved effective.[30]

Lastly, mental health impairment symptoms may be manifested by various behaviors that impede daily interactions, that is, activities of daily living, relationships, and employment, to name a few.[30] A critical care diary is a patient- and family centered approach that could help with stimulation for physical, cognitive, and mental health impairments by filling memory gaps.[24,30] Trends in CAM-ICU can help identify acute changes linked to poor outcomes such as functional decline and potential death.[30]

Management of the Older Adult in Acute Care

Once the geriatric patient transitions from critical care to the acute care environment, the management and goals must be adapted for the new phase of care. The patient's condition has stabilized, and now the aim is prevention of postoperative complications, ongoing rehabilitation to avoid functional decline, and planning for discharge. Because of the unique care requirements of the geriatric population, a multifaceted, interdisciplinary approach is needed. One way to ensure that all elements of care are addressed is to use a geriatric framework. Frameworks for care provide a standardized approach to avoid gaps in care and ensure the needs of the patient are met through a holistic approach.[33]

The use of frameworks and models such as Nurses Improving Care for Healthcare System Elders (NICHE), Acute Care for Elders (ACE), and the IHI 4Ms (see **Fig. 1**) have proved advantageous in decreasing length of stay, preventing readmissions, and decreasing overall cost.[33–36] The CNS is essential in driving the use of frameworks to improve patient outcomes. Although geriatric-specific programs differ slightly, there are similar characteristics that drive a standardized, collaborative approach to patient-centered care. Although all of these programs can increase quality of care, they also require time and funding, which may lead to difficulty garnering leadership support. Commitment to specialized care of the older adult is required to ensure sustainment and success.[33]

Complication Prevention

Prevention of hospital-acquired conditions is important in all postoperative patients. However, the older adult patient is at higher risk for development of complications such as functional decline, infection, or even death.[34] Therefore, complication prevention is an essential part of care for this population. Early recognition and prompt treatment is imperative to prevent mortality and morbidity.

Mobility is one of the most important but often overlooked interventions necessary for prevention of postoperative complications.[34] Bedrest is sometimes used in hospitals due to patient request, for avoidance of falls and to promote rest. Restraints are also used for fall prevention and to manage the symptoms of delirium. Every 1 day spent in bed leads to muscle weakening and degradation that will take three days of mobilizing to recover.[37] Even the act of assisting a patient to a chair for meals can combat functional decline, decrease risk of pulmonary complications, avoid PI, and help regulate the sleep-wake cycle, thereby preventing delirium.[37] Mobilizing the elderly surgical patient as much as their functional ability allows should be made a top priority.

Following surgery and transfer from critical care, the patient will likely have several lines in place such as urinary catheters, central venous intravenous lines, and telemetry. Any invasive line should be removed as soon as possible to decrease infection risk. Even noninvasive lines can pose a risk due to decreased patient mobility related to tethering.[36] The physiologic effects of aging often mean that traditional vital signs and laboratory work may not show the typical signs of infection, especially in frail older adults. Rather, trending results may give an earlier indication of developing infection.[38] Changes in mental status including delirium may also be indicators of new or worsening infection in the older adult. Involving a geriatrician and a CNS in the patient's care team can promote early identification and treatment of complications.[39]

TRANSITION OF CARE FROM ACUTE CARE TO OUTPATIENT

Planning for discharge should ideally begin as soon as a patient is admitted to the hospital, if not sooner.[38,40] The transition from hospital to either home or a skilled nursing facility puts the patient at a high risk for adverse events related to medication errors and miscommunication.[34] Implementation of interventions that standardize the discharge process and support the continuity of care will lead to better outcomes and less readmissions.[40]

Communication Barriers

A patient who is being discharged to home must undergo a thorough assessment so that care can be tailored to meet their needs. Physical ability, social support, cognition, and health literacy should be assessed and paired with the appropriate community resources.[33] The health care team must also assess the patient's physical environment at home to identify any safety concerns or needs. In order to ensure that successful discharge is achieved, the team must involve the patient and family in planning while promoting self-management through education.[41] The essential components of self-management include the ability to recognize reportable symptoms, manage medications and treatments, and coordinate their ongoing care after discharge from the hospital.[42] All discharge instructions and education handouts should be provided to the patient in written format and in their preferred language.[40]

Postdischarge follow-up appointments and telephone check-ins have also been shown to improve outcomes for the geriatric surgical patient.[41] Home health can be an invaluable resource to help the patient manage their care at home and avoid preventable readmission.[34] An innovative solution for navigating the transition from the inpatient to outpatient environment is to engage the CNS in providing longitudinal care by following-up with the patient via phone and in person within the first week after discharge.[43] This approach to transitional care is an effective way to address health equity and bridge communication gaps while providing a billable service.[34,43]

Inpatient provider to outpatient provider communication is another important part of discharge. The discharging physician is responsible for formulating a written handoff to the outpatient provider taking over care. Pending laboratory and radiology studies, recommendations for future studies, and specialist follow-ups should be included in the document.[34] Use of a standardized electronic template can ensure that no elements are missed.[40] In addition, the nurse and provider can collaborate to formulate discharge instructions for a nursing home to make sure that both medical and nursing care continuity is maintained.[33] The CNS can help to coordinate this partnership while providing a holistic lens for discharge planning.[39]

Medication Reconciliation

Medication reconciliation, or lack thereof, at the time of discharge poses a risk for error to all patients. The World Health Organization estimates that up to 80% of patients experience at least one error in medication orders at the time of discharge. Because of the overall complexity of care and number of prescribed medications, older adults are at an even higher risk for adverse medication events than the average hospitalized patient.[40] One proven method to decrease the risk for medication errors is medication reconciliation at discharge using an electronic tool.[41] Because many medications are stopped and started during hospitalization, often related to changing condition and formulary substitutions, it is imperative that medication reconciliation takes place. It can easily become confusing for the older adult when multiple changes to home medications are made, especially if they are receiving automatic refills; this sets the patient up for duplication of therapy and potential adverse health effects. The pharmacist plays an essential role in assuring medication continuity while identifying gaps. Before discharge, the interdisciplinary team should collaborate to complete a thorough review of medications. At minimum, this should include the provider, pharmacist, and CNS.[33,37,39]

SUMMARY

Patient safety is paramount, especially with the high complex and complicated care of this population. With the transition of care in the hospital setting, many risk factors are present in the older adult population. Incorporating the 4Ms for high-quality care sets the patient up for success on the surgical trajectory. Adherence to checklists, frameworks, bundles, and guidelines, along with listening to the patient, enables a safe transition of care throughout the hospital stay for the patient, family, and health care staff. Medical teams with multiple disciplinary approaches with various stakeholders, including trained professionals with adult gerontology, may assist in managing the complex care of the older adult population.

The CNS translates evidence-based practices for standards of care to the bedside with various methods to affect optimal outcomes. CNSs are complex care providers that can be integrated across the patient care continuum, ensuring that the patient, nurses, and system are safe. Timely, clear, and concise communication between health care professionals, along with the patient and family, aids in combatting failures throughout the transition of care. Hand-off through the transition of care is vital; therefore, an integrated, structured approach with optimizing frameworks, bundles, and checklists will set the team and patient up for success and obtain the best outcomes.

CLINICS CARE POINTS

- All older adults should establish an advanced directive before undergoing elective surgery.
- Before a planned surgery, older adults should have a fasting period that allows for clear liquids up to 2 hours before surgery with consideration for those at higher risk for aspiration.
- Older adults are at higher risk for hypothermia in the perioperative phase of care and should be monitored for core temperature maintenance.
- Pressure injury formation in the perioperative period can be avoided by using pressure redistributing surfaces, elevating the heels while supporting the calves, padding bony prominences, and using micro turns when possible

- Use of a comprehensive checklist for routine critical care is recommended.
- Older adults in the critical care environment should have a consult to a geriatrician.
- Patients in critical care should be routinely screened for delirium, and dexmedetomidine may be used if delirium is impeding weaning or extubation from mechanical ventilation.
- As a patient transitions from critical care to acute care, orders for nothing by mouth, restraints, and bedrest should be discontinued as soon as possible.
- The ABCDEF bundle can assist with prevention of postintensive care syndrome.
- Mobilization, nutritional intake, and sleep preservation are interventions that can prevent delirium and promote better patient outcomes.
- Communication failures place the patient and staff at risk for medical errors.
- Approximately 80% of patients experience at least one medication order at the time of discharge.
- Use of a structured handoff with framework or template tools assist with standardization to minimize gaps and improve safety throughout the transitions of care.
- Prevention of postoperative complications is a multifaceted interprofessional approach.
- The older adult population has a higher risk of complications that is, hospital-acquired complications; therefore, use of frameworks improve outcomes and decrease cost that is, length of stay.
- Imperative to monitor trends for postoperative complications.
- Mobility is a top priority and the most important intervention to prevent postoperative complications.
- Remove any invasive line as soon as possible to minimize the risk of infections.
- Tethering devices (ie, noninvasive or invasive) will decrease mobility.
- A standard discharge process leads to better outcomes with less readmissions.
- All discharge instructions or educational handouts to be provided to patients in written format and in their preferred language.
- Postoperative phone call following discharge to be completed within 1 week to assist with the transition of care, address health equity, and bridge communication gaps.
- Providers to use standardized electronic template with discharge outside the hospital to help ensure no elements are missed and minimize errors.

DISCLOSURE

All listed authors do not have any commercial or financial conflicts of interest and/or any funding sources.

REFERENCES

1. Institute of Medicine (US), Committee on quality of health care in America, In: To err is human: building a safer health system, 2000, National Academies Press (US); Washington, DC, 1-2.
2. Institute of Medicine (US). Committee on quality of health care in America. Crossing the quality chasm: a new health system for the 21st century. Washington, DC: National Academies Press (US); 2001.
3. Tsai TC, Joynt KE, Orav EJ, et al. Variation in surgical-readmission rates and quality of hospital care. N Engl J Med 2013;369(12):1134–42.

4. Gupta S, Perry JA, Kozar R. Transitions of care in geriatric medicine. Clin Geriatr Med 2019;35(1):45–52.
5. Riesenberg LA, Leitzsch J, Massucci JL, et al. Residents and attending physicians handoffs: a systematic review of the literature. Acad Med 2009;84(12):1775–87.
6. Gabbard ER, Klein D, Vollman K, et al. Clinical nurse specialist: a critical member of the ICU team. Crit Care Med 2021;49(6):634–41.
7. Scruth EA. Post-intensive care syndrome: preventing complications and improving long- term outcomes. Clin Nurse Spec 2014;28(1):9–11.
8. Beiler J, Opper K, Weiss M. Integrating research and quality improvement using TeamSTEPPS: a health team communication project to improve hospital discharge. Clin Nurse Spec 2019;33(1):22–32.
9. Chow WB, Rosenthal RA, Merkow RP, et al. Optimal preoperative assessment of the geriatric surgical patient: a best practices guideline from the American college of surgeons national surgical quality improvement program and the American geriatrics society. J Am Coll Surg 2012;215(4):453–66.
10. Mohanty S, Rosenthal RA, Russell MM, et al. Optimal perioperative management of the geriatric patient: a best practices guideline from the American College of Surgeons NSQIP and the American Geriatrics Society, J Am Coll Surg, 2016;222(5):930–947.
11. Joshi GP, Abdelmalak BB, Weigel WA, et al. 2023 American Society of Anesthesiologists practice guidelines for preoperative fasting: carbohydrate-containing clear liquids with or without protein, chewing gum, and pediatric fasting duration-A modular update of the 2017 American Society of Anesthesiologists practice guidelines for preoperative fasting, Anesthesiology, 2023;138(2):132–151.
12. Gefen A, Creehan S, Black J. Critical biomechanical and clinical insights concerning tissue protection when positioning patients in the operating room: a scoping review. Int Wound J 2020;17(5):1405–23 [VA] [PubMed: 32496025].
13. Joint Commission on Accreditation of Healthcare Organizations, USA. Using medication reconciliation to prevent errors. Sentinel Event Alert 2006;(35):1–4.
14. Joint Commission on Accreditation of Healthcare Organizations, USA. Inadequate hand- off communication. Sentinel Event Alert 2017;(58):1–6.
15. Rothschild JM, Landrigan CP, Cronin JW, et al. The Critical Care Safety Study: the incidence and nature of adverse events and serious medical errors in intensive care. Crit Care Med 2005;33(8):1694–700.
16. McElroy LM, Collins KM, Koller FL, et al. Operating room to intensive care unit handoffs and the risks of patient harm. Surgery 2015;158(3):588–94.
17. Etzioni DA, Liu JH, Maggard MA, et al. The aging population and its impact on the surgery workforce. Ann Surg 2003;238(2):170–7.
18. Starmer AJ, Spector ND, Srivastava R, et al. Changes in medical errors after implementation of a handoff program. N Engl J Med 2014;371(19):1803–12.
19. Lambert LH, Adams JA. Improved anesthesia handoff after implementation of the written handoff anesthesia tool (WHAT). AANA J (Am Assoc Nurse Anesth) 2018; 86(5):361–70.
20. Lane-Fall MB, Pascual JL, Peifer HG, et al. A partially structured postoperative handoff protocol improves communication in 2 mixed surgical intensive care units: findings from the handoffs and transitions in critical care (HATRICC) prospective cohort study. Ann Surg 2020;271(3):484–93.
21. Pucher PH, Johnston MJ, Aggarwal R, et al. Effectiveness of interventions to improve patient handover in surgery: a systematic review. Surgery 2015;158(1): 85–95.

22. Keller N, Bosse G, Memmert B, et al. Improving quality of care in less than 1 min: a prospective intervention study on postoperative handovers to the ICU/PACU. BMJ Open Qual 2020;9(2):e000668.

23. Lane-Fall MB, Christakos A, Russell GC, et al. Handoffs and transitions in critical care- understanding scalability: study protocol for a multicenter stepped wedge type 2 hybrid effectiveness-implementation trial. Implement Sci 2021;16(1):63.

24. Geen O, Rochwerg B, Wang XM. Optimizing care for critically ill older adults. Canadian Medical Association Journal 2021;193(39). https://doi.org/10.1503/cmaj.210652.

25. Fallon WF Jr, Rader E, Zyzanski S, et al. Geriatric outcomes are improved by a geriatric trauma consultation service. J Trauma 2006;61(5):1040–6.

26. Bradway C, Trotta R, Bixby MB, et al. A qualitative analysis of an advanced practice nurse-directed transitional care model intervention. Gerontol 2012;52(3):394–407.

27. Wissanji T, Forget MF, Muscedere J, et al. Models of care in Geriatric Intensive Care—a scoping review on the optimal structure of care for critically ill older adults admitted in an ICU. Critical Care Explorations 2022;4(4). https://doi.org/10.1097/cce.0000000000000661.

28. Chechel L, McLean B, Slazinski T, et al. What the joint commission medication management titration standards mean to quality care for complex patients. Clin Nurse Spec 2023;37(1):36–41.

29. Kaplow R. Complexity. In: Hardin SR, Kaplow R, editors. Synergy for clinical excellence: the AACN synergy model for patient care. 2nd edition. Burlington, MA: Jones & Bartlett Learning, LLC; 2017. p. 31–5.

30. Brunker LB, Boncyk CS, Rengel KF, et al. Elderly patients and management in intensive care units (ICU): clinical challenges. Clin Interv Aging 2023;18:93–112.

31. O'Hearn PA, Schmidt MM. Facilitating transitions of care. In: Duffy M, Dresser S, Fulton JS, editors. Clinical nurse specialist toolkit: a guide for the new clinical nurse specialist. 2nd edition. New York, NY: Springer Publishing Company; 2016. p. 177–87.

32. Guidet B, Vallet H, Boddaert J, et al. Caring for the critically ill patients over 80: a narrative review. Ann Intensive Care 2018;8(1). https://doi.org/10.1186/s13613-018-0458-7.

33. Enderlin CA, McLeskey N, Rooker JL, et al. Review of current conceptual models and frameworks to guide transitions of care in older adults. Geriatr Nurs 2013;34(1):47–52.

34. Optimal Perioperative Management of the Geriatric Patient: Best Practices Guidelines from ACS NSQIP/American Geriatrics Society. https://www.facs.org/media/y5efmgox/acs-nsqip-geriatric-2016-guidelines.pdf.

35. Capezuti E, Boltz M, Cline D, et al. Nurses Improving Care for Healthsystem Elders - a model for optimising the geriatric nursing practice environment. J Clin Nurs 2012;21(21–22):3117–25. https://doi.org/10.1111/j.1365-2702.2012.04259.x.

36. Age-Friendly Health Systems: Guide to Using the 4Ms in the Care of Older Adults.; 2020. https://www.ihi.org/Engage/Initiatives/Age-Friendly-Health-Systems/Documents/IHIAgeFriendlyHealthSystems_GuidetoUsing4MsCare.pd.

37. Conley DM, Burket TL, Schumacher S, et al. Implementing geriatric models of care: a role of the gerontological clinical nurse specialist—Part I. Geriatr Nurs 2012;33(3):229–34.

38. Quinn TJ, Mooijaart SP, Gallacher K, et al. Acute care assessment of older adults living with frailty. BMJ 2019;31:l13. Published online January.

39. Benedict L, Robinson K, Holder C. Clinical nurse specialist practice within the acute care for Elders interdisciplinary team model. Clin Nurse Spec 2006;20(5): 248–51.
40. Quick Safety Issue 26: Transitions of Care: Managing medications (Updated April 2022). www.jointcommission.org. Accessed March 16, 2023. https://www. jointcommission.org/resources/news-and-multimedia/newsletters/newsletters/ quick-safety/quick-safety-issue-26-transitions-of-care-managing-medications/#. Y9qPonbMKUk.
41. Tomlinson J, Cheong VL, Fylan B, et al. Successful care transitions for older people: a systematic review and meta-analysis of the effects of interventions that support medication continuity. Age Ageing 2020;49(4):558–69.
42. Hladkowicz E, Dumitrascu F, Auais M, et al. Evaluations of postoperative transitions in care for older adults: a scoping review. BMC Geriatr 2022;22(1). https://doi.org/10.1186/s12877-022-02989-6.
43. Allard BL, Conroy CA. Our nursing profession at a crossroads. Nurs Adm Q 2022; 46(3):208–17.

Substance Use Disorder in Critical Care

Monchielle Bolds, MSN, RN, CNE

KEYWORDS

- Substance use disorder • Older • Geriatric • Critical care

KEY POINTS

- Substance use disorders are increasing in the older adult population.
- Risk factors for substance use disorders in the older adult are different from the risk factors for young and middle-aged adults.
- Treating substance use disorders in the older adult ICU patient is complicated by age-related changes and co-morbid conditions.
- Stigma plays a significant role in the therapeutic relationship between the patient and ICU staff and it can prevent the patient from disclosing a substance use disorder.

INTRODUCTION

Substance use disorder (SUD) is a serious problem in the United States (U.S.) and abroad. Critical care nurses are uniquely positioned to address the problem in order to improve patient outcomes. Older adults make up a large portion of the population worldwide and they inevitably make up a large percentage of critical care hospital admissions. The aging baby boomer population has contributed to an increase in older adults.[1] The adult population aged 65 and older has increased by one-third since 2010.[1] The United Nations projects that the population of people aged 65 and older will double by the year 2050.[2] Older adults are admitted to intensive care units (ICU) for acute and chronic illnesses and they are not exempt from experiencing substance use disorders. Substance use disorder in older patients admitted to critical care units can present a host of health and ethical issues.

Definitions

The terms substance use disorder, substance abuse, and addiction are often used interchangeably in the literature. Addiction is defined as the psychological or physical dependence on a substance or behavior.[3] Addiction is a more general term that can include psychological dependence on behaviors such as sex addiction or compulsive gambling.[3] The Diagnostic and Statistical Manual of Mental Disorder 5 (DSM-V) uses

Louisiana State University Health Sciences Center New Orleans, 1900 Gravier Street Office 327, New Orleans, LA 70112, USA
E-mail address: Mbold1@lsuhsc.edu

Crit Care Nurs Clin N Am 35 (2023) 469–479
https://doi.org/10.1016/j.cnc.2023.06.004
0899-5885/23/© 2023 Elsevier Inc. All rights reserved.
ccnursing.theclinics.com

the term substance use disorder (SUD) and defines it as "a cluster of cognitive, behavioral, and physiologic symptoms indicating that the individual continues using the substance despite significant substance-related problems."[4(p483)] Substance use disorder can involve the use of cannabis, alcohol, opioids, hallucinogens, inhalants, sedatives, stimulants, cocaine, anxiolytics, hypnotics, and tobacco, and unknown substances.[4] The DSM-V utilizes a set of criteria to the diagnosis substance use disorder as impaired control, social impairment, risky use, and pharmacologic SUD (**Table 1**).

BACKGROUND
Data

Older adults are not the people that come to mind when most of society thinks of individuals with SUDs, but statistics show that SUDs are on the rise in adults aged 65 and older. A study by Colliver and Gfroerer predicted that marijuana use, illicit drug use, and non-prescription psychotherapeutic drug use will increase exponentially by 2020.[5] Drug overdoses among adults 65 and older have tripled since 2020.[5] Alcohol-related deaths increased by 18% in individuals 65 and older from 2019 to 2020.[5] As with young and middle-aged adults, synthetic opioids such as fentanyl have a devastating effect on people aged 65 and older, with deaths increasing by 53% from 2019 to 2020.[5] Alcohol is the most common substance of abuse, followed by other illicit substances such as marijuana, cocaine, heroin, inhalants, and hallucinogens.[6] Data from the years 2013 to 2015 on older adults revealed a 53.5% increase in treatment seeking for opioid use disorders and the number of heroin users doubled in the same time period.[7] Substance use disorder is a modifiable risk factor for admission to the intensive care unit. A recent study conducted at a hospital in Indianapolis, IN found that about a fourth of all ICU admissions were related to SUD.[8] The research revealed that patients admitted for SUD-related issues had longer durations of hospital stays and higher mortality rates.[8]

Risk Factors

Risk factors for SUD in older adults can differ from young and middle-aged adults due to changing physiologic functions, lifestyle changes, and changing family dynamics. Risk factors include chronic illness and pain, disability, impaired mobility, deteriorating health, grief over the loss of loved ones, loss of a job, reduced income, changes in one's living environment, social isolation, a history of substance use, a history of mental illness, and coping using avoidance behaviors.[9,10] These risk factors are experienced by many older adults and ICU nurses and healthcare providers must be engaged and advocate for patients who are at risk. The aging population of baby boomers and the generations following have a history of experience with substance use and experimentation compared to previous generations.[5] Substance use disorder can contribute to the development and exacerbation of multiple illnesses, but the expectation that the older adult will experience chronic disease and illness may prevent the detection of SUD in the older adult population. The cause of abnormal signs and symptoms that result from SUD in older adults could be mistaken for an acute or chronic illness, or age-related physiologic change.

DISCUSSION
Complications and Concerns of Substance Use Disorder in Critical Care
Increased morbidity
Older adults experience chronic illness and disease more frequently than their younger counterparts. The presence of illness makes it difficult for ICU nurses and providers to

Table 1
DSM-V diagnosis criteria for substance use disorder

Impaired Control	Social Impairment	Risky Use	Pharmacologic
• Individuals need larger amounts of the substance and takes the substance longer than intended • Unsuccessful attempts at abstaining from the substance • Spending most of one's time and effort to obtain, use, and recover after using the substance • Craving of the substance involving the reward system in the brain	• Inability of individuals to fulfill duties, involving, work, family, and other responsibilities • Continued use of the substance despite recurrent negative sequelae • No longer involved in social, work, and recreational activities once previously enjoyed	• Use of the substance in physically unsafe conditions • Continued use of the substance despite it contributing to or causing physical or psychological ailments	• Tolerance • Withdrawal symptoms when the substance is discontinued

differentiate between manifestations of SUD and related illness from the usual diseases that older adults may present with to the ICU. An important component of ICU care often involves treating the cause of an illness. In many cases, it is important to treat the cause of an illness in order for symptoms to resolve.

The older adult experiences many physiologic changes that when combined with the various types of illicit substances, can cause or worsen illness.

The respiratory system in the older adult undergoes changes that result in decreased lung expansion, decreased inflation, and the decreased ability to rid the lungs of foreign particles.[10] The reduced capacity of the lungs is usually only apparent during exertion, however in patients using substances by smoking/inhalation, this can have a worsening effect on the respiratory system. Diseases such as chronic obstructive pulmonary disease and asthma can be caused or exacerbated by using certain illicit substances such as opioids which can cause respiratory depression and hypoxia.[11] The lungs would likely sustain more damage from the chemicals introduced into the lungs via smoking/inhalation.

The cardiovascular system undergoes changes in the aging adult. The heart muscle gradually becomes less efficient and has reduced contractility as individuals age.[10] The older adult is at risk for arrythmias due to a reduction in the number of pacemaker cells.[10] Older adults usually adapt to the changes, while some may experience symptoms during exertion that require a gradual change in activity levels. Threats to the cardiovascular system as a result of substance use include valvular disease, endocarditis, arrhythmias, and hypertension.[10,11] In addition to the illnesses that are associated with SUD, cardiac illnesses such as heart failure can be exacerbated.

The gastrointestinal system in the older adult undergoes changes that include reduced gastric motility, atrophy of intestines, and decreased absorption of fat and vitamins such as B vitamins, vitamin D, and iron.[10] Opioids can contribute to anorexia, chronic constipation, and intestinal obstructions.[11] Alcohol in the older can lead to gastritis, vitamin deficiencies, pancreatitis, liver failure, and malnutrition.[10]

The neurological system of the older person undergoes changes that result in a reduction in cerebral metabolism and blood flow, neurons, and nerve fibers.[10] Alcohol can further damage the neurological system by increasing an individual's risk for dementia with heavy use.[11] Alcohol and other drugs can cause hypertension and place patients at high risk of stroke.[12] Substances of misuse can alter mentation and place the older patient at risk for falls and injuries.

Patients are admitted to the ICU for severe illness and patients with substance use disorders are often sicker with higher rates of mortality.[12] Even when the effects of aging have not been seen, the older adult with substance use disorder will be at risk for liver disease, kidney disease, cardiac disease, falls, memory loss, and motor vehicle accidents.[12] Substance use disorder can affect the older patient's psychological status and sense of well-being. Due to life's changes, some older adults are more isolated and emotionally unstable. Depression, poor self-esteem, and poor-self-confidence are associated with SUD in the older adult.[12]

Withdrawal

Patients who are admitted to the ICU with SUD are at risk for withdrawal symptoms. Withdrawal symptoms are extremely uncomfortable, painful, and can worsen a patient's condition during their ICU stay. Patients with opioid use disorder may relapse simply in an effort to avoid withdrawal symptoms. Opioid withdrawal can occur when ceasing the long-term use of prescription and non-prescription opioids. Opioid withdrawal symptoms are the result of increased norepinephrine release.[13] Patients experience physical symptoms such as muscle aches, abdominal pain, diarrhea, and vomiting that typically last 5 to 10 days.[13] Withdrawal symptoms from opioids are not life threatening in isolation, but when combined with another severe illness, patients can experience illness exacerbations and emotional distress. Nurses and other providers in the ICU may confuse opioid withdrawal symptoms with symptoms of other more common disease processes.

Benzodiazepines are medications that produce a relaxing effect by acting on GABA receptor complexes and inhibiting the process of cellular excitation.[13] Withdrawal symptoms from benzodiazepines can occur in individuals with substance use disorder or individuals taking prescribed benzodiazepines who develop a tolerance. When benzodiazepines are stopped abruptly, individuals may experience anxiety, sleep disturbances, tremors, confusion, palpitations, seizures, and psychosis.[13] Benzodiazepine withdrawal is not life threatening, but the symptoms can last from months to years in patients.[13] The long duration of the physical and psychological symptoms of benzodiazepine withdrawal can negatively affect the older adult and their health outcomes. In the intensive care unit, confusion, sleep disturbances, and seizures can have deleterious effects on patients with other comorbid conditions.

Substance use disorder involving stimulants can cause withdrawal symptoms in older ICU patients if there is an abrupt cessation of intake. The most common stimulant substances of misuse are cocaine and amphetamines.[13] Stimulants act on dopamine and norepinephrine producing excessive alertness and euphoria.[13] Symptoms in patients withdrawing from stimulants involve a pattern of crashing, withdrawal, and extinction.[13] The crashing phase involves a depressed mood, anxiety, and agitation that progresses to increased appetite and fatigue.[13] The withdrawal phase involves the inability to obtain pleasure and reduced energy levels.[13] Extinction occurs when physical cravings resolve, but individuals with SUD involving stimulants may continue to psychologically crave the euphoria produced by the stimulant.[13]

Alcohol withdrawals can be a deadly occurrence in the ICU. Any patient with a SUD involving alcohol is at risk, but the older ICU patient is at an increased risk for injury and death. Alcohol acts on GABA receptors and it results in central nervous system depression.[13] The abrupt cessation of alcohol in individuals who are alcohol dependent, results in central nervous system excitation and overactivity of the autonomic nervous system.[13] Alcohol withdrawal syndrome is the result of the abrupt cessation of alcohol with clinical features occuring in stages.[13] It is important to note that the symptoms of alcohol withdrawal syndrome may not occur in sequence and every symptom may not be experienced by every patient.[14] Alcohol withdrawal syndrome may be interrupted by the intake of alcohol or the administration of medications, but patients may advance to Stage IV if left untreated.[14] Patients with a SUD involving alcohol may experience alcohol withdrawal syndrome even with the reduction of alcohol intake. **Table 2** describes the stages of Alcohol withdrawal syndrome.[13,14]

Pharmacologic Issues

Pharmacologic issues in older patients with a SUD in the ICU are complex. Drug-drug interactions can cause negative sequalae in patients with substance use disorder. Intensive care unit nurses and healthcare providers may not be aware of a patient's substance use history, current substance use, or intoxication while in the hospital. Patients with a history of SUD who are in recovery may refuse pain and anti-anxiety medications when hospitalized in the ICU. They may fear relapsing, but pain and anxiety can negatively affect the disease course and healing. As with all patient with SUDs, older patients with SUD in the ICU for painful conditions may experience inadequate pain control due to tolerance.[15] This may present ICU nurses and providers with complicated decisions to make in which they have to weigh the benefits of giving

Table 2
Alcohol withdrawal syndrome

Stage I 8 h After Last Intake	Stage II 24 h After Last Intake	Stage III 24–48 h After Last Intake	Stage IV 3–12 d After Last Intake
• Increased heart rate	• Tremors	• Tonic-Clonic seizures	• Delirium tremors
• Increased blood pressure	• Insomnia		• Severe confusion
• Tremors may or may not be present	• Diaphoresis		• Severe agitation
• Nausea	• Visual, tactile, auditory hallucinations		• Metabolic abnormalities
• Nervousness	• Insomnia		• Cardiac arrhythmias
	• Nightmares		• Respiratory distress/failure

higher doses of pain medications with the risk of injury to an older patient. Older patients metabolize drugs slower due to the reduced kidney and liver function associated with aging.[9,10] Their brains are more sensitive to drugs and the combination can cause concern for over-sedation resulting in respiratory depression, altered mental status, and abnormal vital signs.[9,10]

Patients in recovery for SUD may be prescribed medications that have side effects that can negatively affect the older patient admitted to the ICU. For example, methadone can cause prolonged QTc and serotonin syndrome.[16] Older patients in the ICU are at an increased risk for arrhythmias as a result of age-related cardiovascular changes, which may be compounded by methadone intake. Common ICU medications such as fluconazole and erythromycin can increase the risk of arrhythmias resulting from prolonged QTc when given in combination with methadone.[16] Methadone, when taken with medications such as tricyclic antidepressants and linezolid, can contribute to serotonin syndrome which can cause diarrhea, agitation, and restlessness.[16]

The intoxication of a patient with alcohol when in the ICU can result in serious injury and illness if combined with commonly used medications. Alcohol is a central nervous system depressant and when combined with benzodiazepines and opioids, patients are at increased risk for falls and respiratory depression.[17] One might wonder how an older ICU patient would become intoxicated with alcohol. Substance use disorder involving alcohol might cause patients to drink alcohol-containing substances such as mouthwash to reduce cravings and symptoms of withdrawal. Alcohol can reduce the responsiveness of certain anti-depressants and when used with monoamine oxidase inhibitors, severe hypertension can occur.[17] Medications such as duloxetine comes with a risk of liver damage and when taken with alcohol the risk is greater.[17] Bupropion is a medication that lowers the seizure threshold. When taken with alcohol, the risk for seizures increases.[17] Substance use disorder involving alcohol increases the risk for bleeding.[17] Patients risk for bleeding increases greatly when alcohol is combined with common ICU medications such as non-steroidal anti-inflammatory medications, and warfarin.[17]

Stigma

Stigma is defined as a characteristic of a person or group that causes them to be discredited by others.[18] People with SUDs may experience health-related stigma which occurs as a result of being diagnosed with a specific health condition.[19] Stigma can lead to discrimination and a lack of empathy toward patients with SUD.[19] Stigma directed at or perceived by an older patient in the ICU with substance use disorder can damage the therapeutic relationship between the nurse and patient. The damaged relationship can result in a lack of transparency about their history. Patients may shy away from telling their health care providers about a SUD fearing poor treatment and judgment from healthcare staff.

RECOMMENDATIONS

Recommendations for care of the older patient with substance use disorder in the ICU involve appropriate assessments, medications, interventions for reducing injury, and interventions for reducing stigma. Assessment tools and a complete patient history are imperative for the facilitation of appropriate care in the older adult with a SUD. Nurses and other health care providers must remember that people of all ages can have a SUD. Stereotyping patients with SUD as being young and middle-aged adults can prevent nurses from even asking about substance use. The recommendations need to address the barriers that hinder older adults from acknowledging that they have a substance use disorder. Patients and nurses may be uncomfortable approaching the subject. According to Tampi and colleagues, "denial of the condition, stigma and/or shame of using addictive substances, reluctance to seek professional help, the lack of financial resources and/or social support, along with insufficient knowledge of SUDs among older individuals are often cited as barriers to appropriate identification and treatment of these disorders."[20(p710)]

Assessment

Assessment tools are important components of determining an older ICU patient's past or present substance use. **Table 3** outlines screening tools for substance use disorders in the older adult.[13,20–22]

Assessing for withdrawal symptoms in the older adult ICU patient with substance use disorder is required to prevent additional medical complications. The clinical opioid withdrawal scale (COWS) is an 11-item scale that can be used in inpatient and outpatient settings.[23] The scale assesses the severity of opioid withdrawals.[23] The Clinical Institute Withdrawal Assessment of Alcohol Scale (CIWA) is a tool that monitors the progression and severity of alcohol withdrawals. The use of these assessment tools can help guide treatment in the older adult admitted to the ICU with SUD.

Pharmacologic

Addressing pharmacologic issues in the older adult ICU patient with substance use disorder involves conducting a complete assessment, monitoring for drug-drug interactions, educating the patient on drug-drug interactions, and obtaining toxicology screening results if warranted. Medications to prevent withdrawals and SUD should be used with caution. Older patients with comorbid conditions must be monitored closely to prevent causing additional health complications. **Table 4** outlines medications that can be used for the prevention of withdrawals and substance use disorder treatment.[11,20,24]

Table 3
Substance use disorder screening tools appropriate for older adults in ICU

Screening Tools	Description	Limitation
Cut down, Annoyed, Guilty, and Eye Opener (CAGE) Adapted to Include Drugs (CAGE-AID)	4 item tool that screens for unhealthy alcohol and drug use.	May not distinguish between active or past drinking
Michigan Alcohol Screening Test-Geriatric Version (MAST-G)	24 questions tool focusing on the risk factors in the older population that may lead to problematic alcohol intake	May not distinguish between active or past drinking
Alcohol Use Disorders Identification Test (AUDIT)/(AUDIT-C)	Audit 10-items/Audit C 3- items Assesses for dangerous alcohol use	Cut off scores for dangerous drinking may need to be changed in different populations and countries
Alcohol, Smoking, and Substance Involvement Screening Test (ASSIST)	8-items tool that assesses for the misuse of prescription drugs	Used in older adults but not validated

Table 4	
Medications used to prevent withdrawal and substance use disorder treatment	
Withdrawal Prevention	**Substance Use Disorder Treatment**
• Clonidine-can be given for tachycardia/ hypertension (opioids/alcohol)	Buprenorphine (opioids)
• Loperamide-diarrhea	Methadone (opioids)
• NSAIDS-pain	Naltrexone (opioids-injection form)
• Trazadone-insomnia	Acamprosate (alcohol)
• Benzodiazepines (alcohol/stimulants)	Disulfiram (alcohol)
• Phenobarbital (alcohol)	Naltrexone (alcohol-pill form)
• Gabapentin (alcohol)	
• Dexmedetomidine (alcohol)	
• Propofol (alcohol)	
• Calcium channel blockers (stimulants)	
• IV ethanol (alcohol)	
• IV hydration (opioids/alcohol) if warranted	
• Thiamine, magnesium, phosphorous, folic acid (alcohol)	
• Carbamazepine (benzodiazepines, alcohol)	

Stigma

Stigma can be reduced by educating ICU nurses, providers, and staff on substance use disorder. Many people believe that people with a SUD are at fault for their disease. They believe that they choose to use drugs, but at the same time they lack self-control. This can create a lack of empathy and lead to stigma.[19] Another way to reduce stigma is to understand that the language used can impact how we view others and how they view themselves. Health care providers should use language that puts the person first when discussing issues of substance use disorder.[11] In addition, refraining from using language that promotes trauma and stigma in patients with substance use disorder goes a long way in preventing stigma and its negative sequalae.[11] These terms include calling someone an addict, junkie, drug seeker, or abuser.[11] The terms "clean" or "dirty" should never be used when discussing patients with substance use disorder. For example, instead of using the term "clean," it would be more appropriate to use the term "abstinent." Instead of using the term "dirty," it would be more appropriate to use the terminology "they tested positive." Instead of using the terms "addict" or "junkie," it would be more appropriate to use the terminology "person with substance use disorder."[11] The words used by ICU nurses and other health care providers can significantly impact how a patient perceives ICU staff, as well as themselves.

SUMMARY

Older adult patients make up a large portion of admits to the intensive care unit. The growing problem and paucity of research on the older population with substance use disorder in the ICU makes the topic an essential one to investigate. Much of the literature on substance use disorder involves young and middle-aged adults. For various reasons, SUDs are missed in older patients in the ICU. Additional research is needed to determine the appropriateness of the current assessment tools for the geriatric population. There are some assessment tools that have been adapted for the older population, but most tools have not. There are not many assessment tools for the presence of SUD and withdrawal symptoms that can be used in the ICU population because patients may be intubated, sedated, and not able to answer questionnaires. The older population has different risk factors for substance use disorder, therefore, risk factor analysis and assessment tools should be catered to the specific population. Increased mortality is a serious concern and the risk of death is compounded in the older adult ICU patient by substance use disorder. Withdrawal symptoms can be avoided but nurses and other healthcare providers need to be aware that substance use disorder is a growing problem in older adults. Identification of substance use disorder and withdrawal symptoms can assist ICU nurses and providers with the implementation of early interventions to prevent the deterioration of the patient's condition. There are medications available to treat withdrawal symptoms and substance use disorder, but the literature is scarce on their use specifically in the older adult population. Finally, attitudes towards patients with substance use disorder impact how care is provided by ICU staff and patient outcomes. It may be beneficial to educate ICU nurses and health care providers on the role of stigma in promoting trauma and poor health outcomes.

CLINICS CARE POINTS

- The increase in substance use disorder in older adult ICU patients will inevitably lead to increased morbidity and mortality.
- Additional research is needed on the various screening tools for substance use disorder and their appropriateness in the older adult ICU patient.
- Withdrawal symptom management in the older adult ICU patient with substance use disorder is an important part of the plan of care, but caution must be used to prevent negative sequalae.
- Interventions for the reduction of stigma toward older adult ICU patients with substance use disorder include education on the harmful effects of stigma and how stigma impacts treatment outcomes in patients with substance use disorder.

DISCLOSURE

The author has nothing to disclose.

REFERENCES

1. 65 and Older Population Grows Rapidly as Baby Boomers Age. United States Census Bureau. https://www.census.gov/programs-surveys/decennial-census/decade/2020/2020-census-main.html. Accessed May 18, 2023.
2. World Population Ageing 2019: Key Messages. United Nations, Department of Economic and Social Affairs. Available at: file:///C:/Users/mbold1/Downloads/WorldPopulationAgeing2019-Report.pdf. Accessed May 18, 2023.
3. Substance use, abuse, and addiction. American Psychological Association Web site. Available at: https://www.apa.org/topics/substance-use-abuse-addiction. Accessed May 16, 2023.
4. Diagnostic and Statistical Manual of Mental Disorders. 5th ed. American Psychiatric Association; 2013. Available at: https://doi-org.ezproxy.lsuhsc.edu/10.1176/appi.books.9780890425596. Accessed May 16, 2023.
5. Colliver JD, Compton WM, Gfroerer JC, et al. Projecting drug use among aging baby boomers in 2020. Ann Epidemiol 2006;16(4):257–65.
6. Mattson M, Lipari R, Hays C, Van Horn, S. A Day in The Life of Older Adults: Substance Use Facts. Available at: https://www.samhsa.gov/data/sites/default/files/report_2792/ShortReport-2792.html. May 11, 2017. Accessed May 17, 2023.

7. Huhn A, Strain E, Tompkins D, et al. A hidden aspect of the U.S. opioid crisis: rise in first-time treatment admission or older adults with opioid use disorder. Drug Alcohol Depend 2018;193:142–7.

8. Westerhausen D, Perkins A, Conley J, et al. Burden of substance abuse-related admissions to the medical ICU. Chest 2020;157(1):61–6.

9. Substance Use in Older Adults. National Institute on Drug Abuse Drug Facts. Updated July 2020. Available at: https://nida.nih.gov/publications/drugfacts/substance-use-in-older-adults-drugfacts. Accessed May 17, 2023.

10. Eliopoulos C. Gerontological nursing. 10th edition. Philadelphia, PA: Wolters Kluwer; 2022.

11. Duggirala R, Khushalani S, Palmer T, et al. Screening for and management of opioid use disorder in older adults in primary care. Clin Geriatr Med 2022;38(1):23–38.

12. Kettaneh A. Substance abuse among the older population: overview and management. J Appl Rehabil Counsel 2015;46(4):11–7.

13. Deshpande R, Gong J, Chadha R, et al. Management of the drug abusing patient in the ICU. In: Kaye A, Vadevelu N, Urman R, editors. Substance abuse: inpatient and outpatient management for every clinician. New York, NY: Springer; 2015. p. 389–406.

14. Carlson RW, Kumar NN, Wong-Mckinstry E, et al. Alcohol withdrawal syndrome. Crit Care Clin 2012;28(4):549–85.

15. Adesoye A, Duncan N. Acute pain management in patients with opioid tolerance. US Pharm 2017;42(3):28–32.

16. Elefritz JL, Murphy CV, Papadimos TJ, et al. Methadone analgesia in the critically ill. J Crit Care 2016;34:84–8.

17. Alcohol-Medication Interactions: Potentially Dangerous Mixes. National Institute on Alcohol Abuse and Alcoholism Website. Available at: https://www.niaaa.nih.gov/health-professionals-communities/core-resource-on-alcohol/alcohol-medication-interactions-potentially-dangerous-mixes Last revised May 6, 2022. Accessed May 15, 2023.

18. Goffman E. Stigma: notes on the management of spoiled identity. Englewood Cliffs, NJ: Prentice Hall; 1963.

19. Brener L, von Hippel W, von Hippel C, et al. Perceptions of discriminatory treatment by staff as predictors of drug treatment completion: utility of a mixed methods approach. Drug Alcohol Rev 2010;29(5):491–7.

20. Tampi R, Tampi D, Elson A. Substance use disorders in the older. Psychiatr Clin 2022;45:707–16.

21. Han B, Moore A. Prevention and screening of unhealthy substance use by older adults. Clinical Geriatric Medicine 2018;34(1):117–29.

22. Sarkar S, Parmar A, Chatterjee B. Substance use disorders in the older: a review. Journal of Geriatric Mental Health. 2015; 26(2): 74-82. Available at: https://www.jgmh.org/text.asp?2015/2/2/74/174271. Accessed May 17, 2023.

23. Wesson DR, Ling W. The clinical opiate withdrawal scale (COWS). J Psychoact Drugs 2003;35(2):253–9.

24. Seshadri A, Appelbaum R, Carmichael SP 2nd, et al. Prevention of alcohol withdrawal syndrome in the surgical ICU: an American association for the surgery of trauma critical care committee clinical consensus document. Trauma Surg Acute Care Open 2022;7(1):e001010. Accessed May, 21, 2023.

Identification and Best Practice Management of Comorbid Geri-Psych Conditions in Critical Care

Noel Koller-Ditto, DNP, APRN, AGCNS-BC

KEYWORDS

- Critical care • Mental health • Psychiatric • Comorbidity • Geri-Psych
- Best practice • Elderly • Suicide

KEY POINTS

- More than half of critical care admissions are older adults with physical and mental illness.
- The prevalence of critically ill patients with psychiatric illness is 2.5 times higher than the general population.
- Health-care professionals are not adequately trained to effectively recognize and treat serious mental illness in elderly.
- Critical care nurses feel ill-prepared to provide the best and safest patient care for patients with mental illness.

INTRODUCTION

Mental and physical illnesses are becoming more symbiotic as comorbidities or multimorbidities. As exemplified by some mental illnesses and associated psychopharmacological treatments associated with increased cardiac and metabolic diseases, as well as the fact that some medical illnesses and associated medications are linked to new or worsening mental health diagnosis. Although this frequent comorbidity affects all age groups, older adults seem to be at greater risk of physical and mental multimorbidity.[1] It is estimated that the world population of 60 years or older will double (2.1 billion) by the year 2050, and those aged 80 years or older, will triple (426 million).[2] As the human body ages, illnesses that were once leading causes of death are now part of the complex and chronic health challenges experienced by those delivering care in the hospital, with more than 50% of critical care admissions for patients aged 65 years or older.[3] As the population of older adults continue to grow, so do those with serious mental illness and health-care professionals that frequently care for geriatric patients that are not adequately educated and trained to effectively recognize and treat serious mental illness.[4]

Eastern Michigan University, College of Nursing, Ypsilanti, MI 48197, USA
E-mail address: nkoller@emich.edu

Crit Care Nurs Clin N Am 35 (2023) 481–493
https://doi.org/10.1016/j.cnc.2023.05.011
0899-5885/23/© 2023 Elsevier Inc. All rights reserved.

ccnursing.theclinics.com

Definitions

Multimorbidity: the presence of 2 or more health conditions.
   Older adult/geriatric: persons age 65 years or older.

BACKGROUND

According to the Centers for Disease Control and Prevention (CDC, 2023), over one in 5 adults in the United States live with a mental illness, and one in 25 live with a serious mental illness (e.g. major depression, bipolar, schizophrenia).[5,6] Consequently, those with depression have a 40% higher risk of developing cardiovascular and metabolic diseases than the general population, and those with serious mental illness are twice as likely to develop these conditions.[7] Furthermore, multimorbidity disproportionally affects older adults (64%) and is associated with adverse outcomes such as decline, distress, frailty, increased use of health care, polypharmacy, treatment burden, and death.[8] The adverse associations between older age, and physical-mental multimorbidity can have implications in critical care.[9]

Mental illnesses are common among critically ill patients admitted to critical care, with studies reporting a prevalence of psychiatric illness approximately 2.5 times that of the general population.[10,11,12] Despite the need for complex critical care plans to be inclusive of patients' comorbid mental health disorders; challenges and constraints exist with identification and treatment. Critical care registered nurses (CCRNs) are trained and well versed in providing highly skilled care to unstable patients with complex life-threating medical illness or disease processes. However, it is not widely known if extensive education focuses on caring for patients with mental illness in the critical care setting. Limitations to this training can leave CCRNs feeling ill-prepared, vulnerable, unsupported, and unable to provide the best and safest possible patient-centered care.[10] Reduced knowledge can also compromise the quality of care delivered toward patients with mental illness. This may be due to actual or perceived stigma and negative attitudes from health-care staff to the patient.[13] A 2020 Harris poll[14] showed that 78% of participants think that mental health and physical health are equally important but only 51% of participants think that physical health is treated as more important than mental health in our current health-care system.

As older adults naturally face fluctuations in their mental, cognitive, and physical health, the relationship among these co-occurring illnesses can escalate a decline in overall health. Interdisciplinary training that includes education not only on mental illness but also on principles of best practice geriatric care can result in safe care of the older adult with complex needs,[15] as well as the reduced use of medications relied on for behavioral support that potentially exacerbate adverse behavioral or medical outcomes.

Due to the aging population compared with the amount of critical care health professionals that are specialized in geriatric care, it has been recommended that incorporating geriatric specific principles often found in acute care for elderly hospital units would be most pragmatic to incorporate into critical care standards of the elderly.[16] Some of the suggested practices is to implement best practice bundles and minimize the use of restraints and tethers for delirium prevention, screen for symptoms of depression with prolonged admissions, and pharmacist collaboration for daily reviews of medications including those that are high-risk (sedatives, opioids, and antipsychotics) to minimize inappropriate polypharmacy.[16] This article discusses 4 familiar mental health conditions in older adults present in the critical care environments; psychosis, delirium, depression, and suicide.

DISCUSSION
Psychosis

It is not uncommon for older adults to experience a psychotic episode later in life because of complex interactions (biological, social, environmental, and psychological).[17] Psychotic disorders can present with different clinical features because there are multiple causes, and the presence of psychotic disorders is associated with morbidity and mortality among older adults.[17,18] Potential causes for psychosis can be a result of primary factors such as schizophrenia, schizoaffective disorder, depression, bipolar, dementia, or a result of secondary factors such as substance abuse, delirium, medications, and underlying medical conditions.[17] Psychosis co-occurring in the critical care environment is often referred to as "ICU (Intensive Care Unit) psychosis" and is the result of delirium.

Identification and assessment

Identification of psychosis can be seen through clinical observation of delusions, hallucinations, disorganized motor movements, behavior, or thinking.[19] To determine appropriate treatment, it is imperative that when psychosis is suspected or identified, a comprehensive evaluation should be completed (**Fig. 1**) to identify potential causes and differential diagnoses considering patient age, and history components such as timing of symptoms, earlier medical history, family history, and symptoms stemming from physical, psychiatric, or neurologic cause.[20] Psychosis itself is not a diagnosable disease but a set of symptoms seen with psychotic disorders. The confirmation of psychosis is not through testing but through clinical findings.[20]

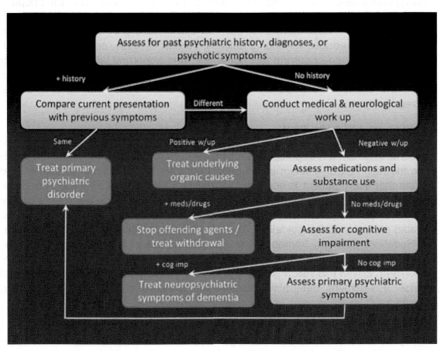

Fig. 1. Etiology assessment of psychosis. (*From* Tampi, et. Al, 2019. Pathway for identifying the etiologies for psychotic symptoms in late life. (**Figure 1** in original).

Therapeutic options
Best practice treatment of psychosis in the older patient should focus on nonpharmacological management strategies and the development of a comprehensive, collaborative, and person-centered treatment plan focused on the underlying cause.[21] Collaborative care teams may include a pharmacist, geriatrician, and psychiatrist. Psychopharmacology treatments using antipsychotics should be used cautiously, judiciously, and with regular monitoring of risk versus benefit. For example, the treatment of agitation and psychosis with antipsychotics should be reserved for emergency use when the symptoms are severe and placing significant distress or danger to the patient.[21] Because the older patient is at higher risk for pharmacological side effects, initiating psychotropic medications should be done with the "low and slow" method, with the initial dosing as low as possible and with slow titration whenever possible.[22] Use of antipsychotics in geriatric patients is associated with increased risks in cerebrovascular events, metabolic side effects, prolonged QT interval measurment on an electrocardiogram, pneumonia, and death.[23] The American Geriatrics Society Beers Criteria for potentially inappropriate medication use in older adults can provide best practice guidance on medication avoidance in elderly patients.[24]

Delirium

Although it is common (up to 80%) for patients to develop delirium in the critical care setting, it can often be under recognized and diagnosed, which leads to delayed or inappropriate treatment of the cause.[25,26] Clinical features of delirium seen in hospitalized patients may include altered attention and cognition, and can include hyper (increased psychomotor, agitation, mood changes) or hypo (reduced psychomotor activity) characteristics.[27] When older patients experience delirium in the hospital, it is met with mutually negative outcomes for the patient, their loved ones, and health-care staff.[28] Risk factors for delirium can include predisposing (older age, men, dementia, reduced functional abilities, cardiac disease, sepsis, hearing and/or vision deficits, co-occurring alcohol abuse, and abnormal laboratory values) or precipitating (drugs, medications, surgery, respiratory failure, prolonged mechanical ventilation, immobility, impaired sleep, acute pain, infections, and illnesses) causes.[29,30]

Identification and assessment
Because nearly 40% of delirium cases are deemed preventable, and delirium can be a clinical emergency, it is imperative that bedside clinical recognition occurs.[27] Considering the high risk of delirium in the critical care setting, standards of care should include that every patient is screened for delirium, using a valid tool, by the nurse once per shift and at anytime there is clinical suspicion.[31] The Confusion Assessment Method for the ICU (CAM-ICU) is one of the 2 recommended screening tools from the updated clinical practice guidelines for Prevention and Management of Pain, Agitation/Sedation, Delirium, Immobility, and Sleep Disruption in Adult Patients in the ICU,[32] and also supported by the Hartford Institute for Geriatric Nursing.[33] A positive screen (**Fig. 2**) with this validated tool should be followed by a comprehensive clinical provider assessment, determining the underlying cause, and swiftly begin treating such cause.[31]

Therapeutic options
Antipsychotic use for delirium is no longer supported as a routine treatment of those that are critically ill, and there continues to be no gold standard medication that is arguably effective.[30] Nonpharmacological approaches to manage delirium in the

CAM-ICU Worksheet

Feature 1: Acute Onset or Fluctuating Course	Score	Check here if Present
Is the patient different than his/her baseline mental status? OR Has the patient had any fluctuation in mental status in the past 24 h as evidenced by fluctuation on a sedation/level of consciousness scale (i.e., RASS/SAS), GCS, or previous delirium assessment?	Either question Yes →	☐
Feature 2: Inattention		
Letters Attention Test (See training manual for alternate **Pictures**) Directions: Say to the patient, *"I am going to read you a series of 10 letters. Whenever you hear the letter 'A,' indicate by squeezing my hand."* Read letters from the following letter list in a normal tone 3s apart. **S A V E A H A A R T** or **C A S A B L A N C A** or **A B A D B A D A A Y** **Errors are counted when patient fails to squeeze on the letter "A" and when the patient squeezes on any letter other than "A."**	Number of Errors >2 →	☐
Feature 3: Altered Level of Consciousness		
Present if the Actual RASS score is anything other than alert and calm (zero)	RASS anything other than zero →	☐
Feature 4:Disorganized Thinking		
Yes/No Questions (See training manual for alternate set of questions) 1. Will a stone float on water? 2. Are there fish in the sea? 3. Does one pound weigh more than two pounds? 4. Can you use a hammer to pound a nail? **Errors are counted when the patient incorrectly answers a question.** **Command** Say to patient: "Hold up this many fingers" (Hold 2 fingers in front of patient) "Now do the same thing with the other hand" (Do not repeat number of fingers) *If the patient is unable to move both arms, for 2nd part of command ask patient to "Add one more finger" **An error is counted if patient is unable to complete the entire command.**	Combined number of errors >1→	☐

Overall CAM-ICU	Criteria Met →	☐ CAM-ICU Positive (Delirium Present)
Feature 1 plus 2 and either 3 or 4 present = CAM-ICU positive	Criteria Not Met →	☐ CAM-ICU Negative (No Delirium)

Fig. 2. CAM-ICU screen. (*From* Copyright © 2002, E. Wesley Ely, MD, MPH and Vanderbilt University, all rights reserved with permission. Resources and tools can be found at: https://www.icudelirium.org/medical-professionals/delirium/monitoring-delirium-in-the-icu.)

critical care patient is the foundational approach supported by the Society of Critical Care Medicine.[30] The most widely used approach has focused on prevention with the ABCDE bundle (awakening and breathing coordination, delirium monitoring/management, and early exercise/mobility), which has been shown to significantly reduce delirium. The current/revised bundle includes a change to "A" for the assessment and treatment of pain, and the inclusion of "F" for family engagement.[34] The new bundle (**Fig. 3**), referred to as the ICU Liberation Bundle (A–F) by the Society of Critical Care Medicine, has shown success to reduce hospital death by 68%, reduce delirium by 25% to 30%, and reduce physical restraints by 60% or more.[35] When delirium does develop, and quickly after identification, the provider assessment can quickly evaluate

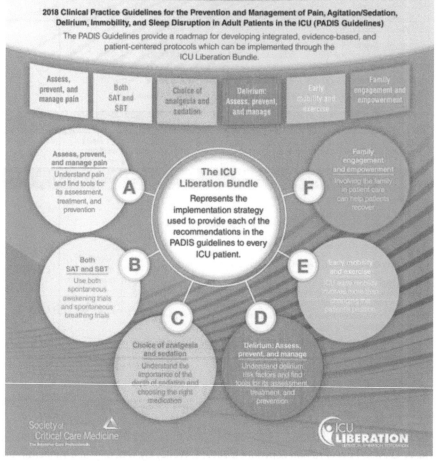

Fig. 3. ICU liberation bundle (A–F). (*From* ICU Liberation Bundle (A–F). Society of Critical Care Medicine.)

factors that may be causing the delirium. In the older adult, there is often more than one etiological factor, and most are treatable, nonbrain disorders.[29] There are several mnemonics found in the literature that are used to determine differential diagnoses and recommended treatment of etiology.[36]

Depression

Depression among older adults is the most prevalent mental health problem they face and is linked to distress, suffering, and impairments with functioning (physical, mental, and social). Often misconceived to be a normal part of aging, depressive disorders in the elderly remain widely underrecognized or un/under treated. This has adverse affects on the course and treatment of other chronic diseases; increases visits to the doctor and emergency room, and use of medications, and impacts longer lengths of stay in the hospital.[5] There are significant groups of critical care patients that have preexisting mental health illnesses, particularly depression. Additionally, it is known that preexisting mental health illnesses are associated with increased mortality post-ICU discharge, making accurate identification and timely treatment essential for the patient's course of care.[37]

Identification and assessment

Although there may be a multitude of screening tools for depression, few are created specifically for older adults. The geriatric depression scale (GDS) is the most widely used tool, with the short form (**Fig. 4**) easily used with medical illness and mild to moderately cognitively impaired older adults.[38] All too often in the acute care environment, depression is seen as an outpatient issue, not as a contributory factor to other disease processes or management. For a positive depression screen, it is essential that a standardized response protocol be implemented to evaluate the patient further. Additionally, because efficacy of the medication can take up to 2-months, it is much easier to begin collaborative care with recognition versus the risk of it being

MOOD SCALE
(short form)

Choose the best answer for how you have felt over the past week:

1. Are you basically satisfied with your life? YES / **NO**

2. Have you dropped many of your activities and interests? **YES** / NO

3. Do you feel that your life is empty? **YES** / NO

4. Do you often get bored? **YES** / NO

5. Are you in good spirits most of the time? YES / **NO**

6. Are you afraid that something bad is going to happen to you? **YES** / NO

7. Do you feel happy most of the time? YES / **NO**

8. Do you often feel helpless? **YES** / NO

9. Do you prefer to stay at home, rather than going out and doing new things? **YES** / NO

10. Do you feel you have more problems with memory than most? **YES** / NO

11. Do you think it is wonderful to be alive now? YES / **NO**

12. Do you feel pretty worthless the way you are now? **YES** / NO

13. Do you feel full of energy? YES / **NO**

14. Do you feel that your situation is hopeless? **YES** / NO

15. Do you think that most people are better off than you are? **YES** / NO

Answers in **bold** indicate depression. Although differing sensitivities and specificities have been obtained across studies, for clinical purposes a score > 5 points is suggestive of depression and should warrant a follow-up interview. Scores > 10 are almost always depression.

Fig. 4. Geriatric depression scale: short form. From: https://web.stanford.edu/~yesavage/GDS.html. This scale is public domain.

overlooked during the course of step-down and discharge care. Considering that the critical care environment may not always present the opportunity to implement screening tools; it should be noted that if the older patient is displaying signs or symptoms of depression, a response by the health-care team should be just the same. Depression is one of the most successfully treated illnesses, but the neglect to identify and treat, can lead to decreases in quality of life and an increase in physical and cognitive impairment. Depression is a common precipitant of suicidal ideation and behavior and the most common diagnosis among those who die by suicide.[38,39]

Therapeutic options

First-line pharmacologic treatment of depression in the criticaly ill patient is the use of low-dose monotherapy with atypical antidepressants, selective serotonin reuptake inhibitors, or serotonin norepinephrine reuptake inhibitors, with the last 2 increasingly supported for use in the older patient.[40] Considerations should include continuing patient's home antidepressants to avoid risky complications from abrupt cessation; however, in the presence of delirium or risky medication interactions, cessation may need to be considered.[40] Further geriatric considerations should include calculations of risk such as a clear medication reconciliation as many older adults may have a trial history of pharmacological treatments that have worked, and not worked; thorough education to the patient and/or caregiver with proven understanding to the reason for use and importance of medication compliance; adherence to follow-up appointments and reporting of negative effects from the antidepressants.[41] As previously discussed, the use of a collaborative care team can assist with reccomendations for use of, or pausing, medication regimens.

Suicide

Suicide is a complex health issue and affects all age groups. Suicide risk among older adults is both alarming and has higher rates than younger age groups, yet not as widely discussed or acknowledged in the medical setting. Vital data shows that adults aged 75 years and older have one of the highest rates of suicide(20.3 per 100,000) in the United States, men aged 75 and older have the highest rate (42.2 per 100,000), adults carefully plan and carry out more deadly suicide attempts, are less likely to be rescued or found, and are less likely to recover from a suicide attempt.[42,43] Suicide risk in the United States is a serious public health problem, and every area of our hospitals has opportunities to play a part in prevention, including the critical care units which have nearly one-third of admissions from patients post suicide attempt.[44] Risk factors for elderly suicide include depression and other chronic illnesses and pain, prior suicidal attempts, impulsivity mixed with cognitive impartment, recent losses, alcohol abuse, and access to lethal means, especially guns and medication.[42] Warning signs of an older adult thinking about suicide include acute personality changes, loss of interest in what used to provide joy, suddenly changing end-of-life wishes, socially avoidant, self-care neglect, fixated with death, and making overt suicidal statements.[42,45]

Identification and assessment

The critical care environment cares for not only patients after a suicide attempt, but also patients who are at risk for suicide and who may not have been yet identified as at risk. This creates 2 important objectives, identify patients who may be at risk, and keep patients identified at high risk for suicide safe while receiving critical care. Identification of patients at risk for suicide can be done using a validated screening tool or through direct statements or behavior displayed by the patient. References for validated/evidenced-based suicide screening tools can be found in the *Suicide Prevention Resources to support Joint Commission Accredited organizations implementation of NPSG 15.01.01.*[46]

Competent identification and assessment of suicide requires increasing the skilled knowledge and awareness among non-psychiatric nurses, including the critical care environment. All patients that are identified to be at risk for suicide need to be evaluated by a clinical professional that is trained to assess the overall risk of suicide and formulate a plan of care to mitigate the risk of self-harm within the hospital, and focuses on safety after discharge.[47]

Therapeutic options

In addition to managing critical medical needs, the top priority when caring for a patient identified at risk for suicide is to protect them from self-harm. Hospital policies written for care and observation of the patient at risk for suicide should always include critical care units. For ongoing management of psychiatric needs, including after suicide attempts and identified suicide risk, consultation to Psychiatry should be included early in the plan of care.[44] In a review of literature[48] on preventing elderly suicide, a key theme found was an early recognition and referral for help/treatment. Whether in the community or the hospital setting, the steps for prevention should align. Identification of any risk for suicide should not be taken lightly or dismissed because of the critical care focus. Plans of care should be clearly written in the patients' medical record and continue through step-down care and/or discharge because the height of suicide risk can be increased after discharge. Best practice inclusions are engaging the patient in the plan of care, creating a safety plan, reducing access to lethal means, and supporting strong handoffs.[49]

SUMMARY

Older patients are vulnerable, as is populations of those with mental illness. Collectively, these vulnerabilities, combined with critical illness, places the older patient at risk for poorer outcomes and death. Especially when comorbid mental illness is underdiagnosed and treated. Physical-mental health multimorbidity continues to increase, the older population continues to live longer, and the combination of both creates vulnerabilities in hospitals, especially within nurses providing care to these patients. When there continues to be a lack of education, knowledge, and clinical processes to address the care of patients with mental health comorbidities, it decreases nurses' confidence and satisfaction. When nurses are repeatedly faced with situations that make them feel as if they cannot provide quality care, dissatisfaction can lead to burnout, and burnout contributes to the critical shortage health-care systems are facing.

Hospitals can reduce these burdens by creating critical care policies and practices that are inclusive of geriatric and mental health concepts, care, and continuing education to those providing care. Standardized approaches should include signs/symptoms of commonly experienced mental health illnesses, best practice screenings and assessments, best practice nonpharmacologic approaches to prevent and treat, and safe practice standards for pharmacologic approaches. Development of best practice policies should be informed through multidisciplinary specialists and should include role delineation (eg, Who can screen, who can assess, what will consultants do). Physical-mental health multimorbidity is the new face of health care for all units, and hospitals need to bridge gaps in not just care but education to see positive outcomes for patients and nurses.

CLINICS CARE POINTS

- Critical care standards should include geriatric best practice principles: minimize the use of restraints, screen for depression, and perform daily reviews of high-risk medications.

- Identify the underlying cause when psychosis is present in elderly. Best practice treatment of psychosis in the older patient should focus on nonpharmacological management strategies and the development of a comprehensive, collaborative, and person-centered treatment plan.
- Without mental health inclusive training, critical care nurses feel vulnerable and unsupported to provide the best and safest possible patient-centered care to patients with mental illness.
- Up to 40% delirium can be prevented. The best practice intervention includes the use of the ABCDE bundle, now referred to as the ICU Liberation Bundle (A–F).
- Depression among older adults is the most prevalent mental health problem they face yet remains widely underrecognized and un/under treated.
- Preexisting mental health illness is associated with increased mortality post-ICU discharge.
- Men aged 75 years and older have the highest rate of suicide in the United States.
- Older adults carry out more deadly suicide attempts and are less likely to recover from a suicide attempt.
- Validated screening tools should be implemented into workflows for mental health conditions: CAM-ICU (delirium), GDS-short form (depression), and refer to Suicide Prevention Resources to support Joint Commission Accredited organizations implementation of NPSG 15.01.01[39] for validated/evidenced-based suicide screening tools.
- Antipsychotic use in the elderly should be cautioned and follow the "slow and low" principles if used.

DISCLOSURE

There are no commercial or financial conflicts of interest to disclose.

REFERENCES

1. Arokiasamy P, Uttamacharya U, Jain K, et al. The impact of multimorbidity on adult physical and mental health in low- and middle-income countries: what does the study on global ageing and adult health (SAGE) reveal? BMC Med 2015;13(1). https://doi.org/10.1186/s12916-015-0402-8.
2. World Health Organization. Mental health of older adults. Who.int. Published 2017. Available at: https://www.who.int/news-room/fact-sheets/detail/mentalhealth-of-older-adults. Accessed January 18, 2023.
3. Miniksar ÖH, Özdemir M. Clinical features and outcomes of very elderly patients admitted to the intensive care unit: a retrospective and observational study. Indian J Crit Care Med 2021;25(6):629–34.
4. Older adults living with serious mental illness. Available at: https://store.samhsa.gov/sites/default/files/d7/priv/pep19-olderadults-smi.pdf. Accessed March 30, 2023.
5. CDC. The State of Mental Health and Aging in America.; 2018. Available at: https://www.cdc.gov/aging/pdf/mental_health.pdf. Accessed March 20, 2023.
6. Centers for Disease Control and Prevention. About mental health. Centers for Disease Control and Prevention. Published June 28, 2021. Available at: https://www.cdc.gov/mentalhealth/learn/index.htm. Accessed February 5, 2023.
7. National Alliance on Mental Illness. Mental health by the numbers. NAMI. Published June 2022. Available at: https://www.nami.org/mhstats. Accessed March 20, 2023.

8. Cheng GJ, Wagner AL, O'Shea BQ, et al. Multimorbidity and mental health trajectories among middle-aged and older US adults during the COVID-19 pandemic: longitudinal findings from the COVID-19 coping study. Innovation in Aging 2022. https://doi.org/10.1093/geroni/igac047.

9. Lee SH, Lee TW, Ju S, et al. Outcomes of very elderly (80 years) critical-ill patients in a medical intensive care unit of a tertiary hospital in Korea. Kor J Intern Med 2017;32(4):675–81.

10. Weare R, Green C, Olasoji M, et al. ICU nurses feel unprepared to care for patients with mental illness: a survey of nurses' attitudes, knowledge, and skills. Intensive Crit Care Nurs 2019;53:37–42.

11. Mahmoodimeymand A. A review of the prevalence of mental disorders in intensive care units in hospitals: review study. International Journal of Hospital Research 2023;12(1). http://ijhr.iums.ac.ir/article_139886.html. Accessed April 8, 2023.

12. Cobert J, Jeon SY, Boscardin J, et al. Trends in geriatric conditions among older adults admitted to US ICUs between 1998 and 2015. Chest 2022;161(6): 1555–65.

13. Zahid M, Al-Awadhi A, Atawneh F, et al. Nurses' attitude towards patients with mental illness in a general hospital in Kuwait. Saudi Journal of Medicine and Medical. Sciences 2017;5(1):31.

14. National Public Perception of Mental Health and Suicide Prevention Survey Results | National Action Alliance for Suicide Prevention. theactionalliance.org. Available at: https://theactionalliance.org/resource/national-public-perception-mental-health-and-suicide-prevention-survey-results. Accessed March 16, 2021.

15. Brunker LB, Boncyk CS, Rengel KF, et al. Elderly patients and management in intensive care units (ICU): clinical challenges. Clin Interv Aging 2023;18:93–112.

16. Geen O, Rochwerg B, Wang XM. Optimizing care for critically ill older adults. CMAJ (Can Med Assoc J) 2021;193(39):E1525–33.

17. Tampi RR, Young J, Hoq R, et al. Psychotic disorders in late life: a narrative review. Therapeutic Advances in Psychopharmacology 2019;9. https://doi.org/10.1177/2045125319882798.

18. Byrne P. Managing the acute psychotic episode. BMJ 2007 Mar 31;334(7595): 686–92.

19. Maj M, van Os J, De Hert M, et al. The clinical characterization of the patient with primary psychosis aimed at personalization of management. World Psychiatr 2021;20(1):4–33.

20. Vyas CM, Petriceks AH, Paudel S, et al. Acute psychosis: differential diagnosis, evaluation, and management. Prim Care Companion CNS Disord 2023;25(2): 22f03338.

21. Reus VI, Fochtmann LJ, Eyler AE, et al. The American psychiatric association practice guideline on the use of antipsychotics to treat agitation or psychosis in patients with dementia. Am J Psychiatr 2016;173(5):543–6.

22. Varma S, Sareen H, Trivedi JK. The geriatric population and psychiatric medication. Mens Sana Monogr 2010;8(1):30–51.

23. Rogowska M, Thornton M, Creese B, et al. Implications of adverse outcomes associated with antipsychotics in older patients with dementia: a 2011–2022 update. Drugs Aging 2023;40:21–32.

24. American Geriatrics Society. American geriatrics society 2019 updated AGS beers criteria for potentially inappropriate medication use in older adults. J Am Geriatr Soc 2019;67(4). https://doi.org/10.1111/jgs.15767.

25. Clinic Cleveland. Delirium and mental confusion: symptoms, causes, treatment & prevention. Cleveland Clinic; 2020. Available at: https://my.clevelandclinic.org/health/diseases/15252-delirium. Accessed March 30, 2023.

26. Park SY, Lee HB. Prevention and management of delirium in critically ill adult patients in the intensive care unit: a review based on the 2018 PADIS guidelines. Acute Crit Care 2019;34(2):117–25.

27. Johansson YA, Bergh I, Ericsson I, et al. Delirium in older hospitalized patients—signs and actions: a retrospective patient record review. BMC Geriatr 2018;18:43.

28. Balas MC, Rice M, Chaperon C, et al. Management of delirium in critically ill older adults. Crit Care Nurse 2012;32(4):15–26.

29. Marcantonio ERMD. Delirium in hospitalized older adults. N Engl J Med 2017; 377:1456–66.

30. Mart MF, Williams Roberson S, Salas B, et al. Prevention and management of delirium in the intensive care unit. Semin Respir Crit Care Med 2021;42(1):112–26.

31. Miranda F, Arevalo-Rodriguez I, Díaz G, et al. Confusion Assessment Method for the intensive care unit (CAM-ICU) for the diagnosis of delirium in adults in critical care settings. Cochrane Database Syst Rev 2018;2018(9):CD013126.

32. Devlin JW, Skrobik Y, Gélinas C, et al. Clinical Practice Guidelines for the Prevention and Management of Pain, Agitation/Sedation, Delirium, Immobility, and Sleep Disruption in Adult Patients in the ICU. Crit Care Med 2018;46(9):e825–73.

33. Tate J, Balas M. general assessment series Best Practices in Nursing Care to Older Adults The Confusion Assessment Method for the ICU (CAM-ICU). doi:https://doi.org/10.1016/j.aucc.2011.01.002.

34. Marra A, Ely EW, Pandharipande PP, et al. The ABCDEF Bundle in Critical Care. Crit Care Clin 2017;33(2):225–43.

35. Grieshop S. ABCDEF bundle. Am J Crit Care 2023;32(2):100.

36. Terminology & Mnemonics. www.icudelirium.org. https://www.icudelirium.org/medical-professionals/terminology-mnemonics.

37. Pilowsky JK, Elliott R, Roche MA. Pre-existing mental health disorders in patients admitted to the intensive care unit: a systematic review and meta-analysis of prevalence. J Adv Nurs 2021. https://doi.org/10.1111/jan.14753.

38. The Geriatric Depression Scale (GDS). Available at: https://hign.org/sites/default/files/2020-06/Try_This_General_Assessment_4.pdf. Accessed March 4, 2023.

39. PATIENT SAFETY SCREENER (PSS-3) and TIP SHEET. Available at: https://sprc.org/wp-content/uploads/2022/11/Patient-Safety-Screener-PSS-3-and-Tip-Sheet.pdf. Accessed March 8, 2023.

40. Beach Scott R, Stern Theodore A. Antidepressants in critical illness. In: Webb Andrew, others, editors. Oxford textbook of critical care. 2 edition. Oxford: Oxford Academic; 2016. https://doi.org/10.1093/med/9780199600830.003.0044. Accessed 7 April. 2023.

41. Lenze EJ, Ajam Oughli H. Antidepressant treatment for late-life depression: considering risks and benefits. J Am Geriatr Soc 2019;67(8):1555–6.

42. National Council on Aging. The National Council on Aging. ncoa.org. Published 2022. Available at: https://ncoa.org/article/suicide-and-older-adults-what-you-should-know. Accessed February 5, 2023.

43. CDC. Disparities in Suicide. Available at: https://www.cdc.gov/suicide/facts/disparities-in-suicide.html. Accessed June 22, 2023.

44. Phadke S, Marwale A, Kocher A. Psychiatric management of patients in intensive care units. Indian J Psychiatr 2022;64(8):292.

45. Preventing Suicide in Older Adults. Mental Health America. Available at: https://www.mhanational.org/preventing-suicide-older-adults#:~:text=Risk%20Factors

%20and%20Warning%20Signs&text=Prior%20suicide%20attempts.   Accessed April 8, 2023.

46. SELECTION of RESOURCES. https://www.jointcommission.org/standards/national-patient-safety-goals/-/media/83ac7352b9ee42c9bda8d70ac2c00ed4.ashx.

47. National Patient Safety Goal for Suicide Prevention; 2019. https://www.joint commission.org/-/media/tjc/documents/standards/r3-reports/r3_18_suicide_ prevention_hap_bhc_cah_11_4_19_final1.pdf.

48. Holm AL, Salemonsen E, Severinsson E. Suicide prevention strategies for older persons—an integrative review of empirical and theoretical papers. Nursing Open 2021. https://doi.org/10.1002/nop2.789.

49. Framework | Zero Suicide. zerosuicide.edc.org. Available at: https://zerosuicide.edc.org/about/framework. Accessed March 3. 2023.

A Team Approach to Bundle Compliance

Joseph Eppling, DNP, MHA, RN, CRRN, NEA-BC[a],*,
Rachel Nickel, BSN, MBA, RN, CCRN[b]

KEYWORDS

- Ventilator-associated pneumonia (VAP) • Ventilator-associated events (VAEs)
- Health care-associated infection (HAI) • Prevention • Bundles

KEY POINTS

- Hospitals aim to enhance patient care and prevent hospital-acquired conditions (HACs) such as ventilator-associated pneumonia (VAP).
- There are currently no established standards for preventing VAP, and no single element that directly addresses VAP prevention.
- Evidence consistently supports the use of bundled care, incorporating multiple interventions, as the most effective approach to reduce or eliminate VAP.
- A quality improvement project was undertaken, involving an interprofessional team, to assess current practices and compare them with evidence-based practices in the literature.
- This project resulted in the development and implementation of a critical care VAP bundle practice, which led to both improved compliance with bundled care and improved VAP rates.

INTRODUCTION

Health-care organizations across the country are focused on quality and patient outcomes. Concentration on improving outcomes is not only the right thing to do but also reimbursement and funding are directly tied to the facilities' outcome measures. A major emphasis on quality has been focused toward reducing hospital-acquired conditions (HACs). According to the Agency for Healthcare Research and Quality (AHRQ), a HAC is a condition that occurs during a hospital stay whereby the patient was not being treated for the condition during admission and therefore is considered

[a] Louisiana State University Health Science Center School of Nursing, 1900 Gravier Street, New Orleans, LA 70112, USA; [b] University Medical Center New Orleans, 2000 Canal Street, New Orleans, LA 70118, USA
* Corresponding author.
E-mail address: jeppli@lsuhsc.edu

Crit Care Nurs Clin N Am 35 (2023) 495–504
https://doi.org/10.1016/j.cnc.2023.06.005
0899-5885/23/© 2023 Elsevier Inc. All rights reserved.
ccnursing.theclinics.com

preventable. These conditions can cause harm to patients and hospitals are actively attempting to prevent and reduce HAC. Ventilator-associated pneumonia (VAP) is one such event.[1] A VAP is defined as a patient on a ventilator for more than 48 hours and diagnosed with pneumonia. Unfortunately, VAP as an HAC, is one of the leading causes of death, and is considered the most common HAC in critical care units.[2] In 2013, the Center for Disease Control and Prevention (CDC) began defining other respiratory conditions when patients are mechanically ventilated as ventilator-associated events (VAEs) other than pneumonia due to the difficulty in defining VAP and the many definitions. There are currently 3 definitions that define VAE and include ventilator-associated conditions, infection-related ventilator-associated complication, and possible VAP. These are also conditions that are considered avoidable.[3] Patients admitted to a critical care unit that are on a ventilator and are immunocompromised, elderly, and/or postoperative are more at risk and have higher rates of infection such as VAP.[4]

BACKGROUND

This quality improvement project took place at a large academic medical center in Southeast Louisiana in the intensive care units (ICUs). The facility is one hospital that is part of a larger health-care system with other acute care hospitals. This hospital is licensed for 446 acute care beds. Of the total beds, 48 are critical care beds encompassing 24 medical intensive care unit (MICU) beds and 24 trauma intensive care unit (TICU) beds. Both ICUs admit greater than 2400 patients each annually with an average daily census between 18 and 20, respectively. The ICUs participate in the organization's Critical Care Committee as part of the shared governance structure. The Critical Care Committee meets every other month and includes medical staff and nursing representation from all critical care areas including MICU, TICU, Emergency Department, and the Burn Center. In addition, other departments that support critical care attend the committee meeting including respiratory, pharmacy, infection control, and quality. The Critical care committee has several functions and responsibilities that include but are not limited to reviewing, recommending, and/or developing critical care policies and protocols, reviewing quality metrics, establishing goals, and discussing departmental action plans and progress along with other duties. During the July 2022 meeting, it was noted that both the MICU and TICU units continued to improve with nursing sensitive measures, even throughout the coronavirus disease 2019 (COVID-19) pandemic. However, metrics regarding VAP did not demonstrate any substantial improvements and discussion ensued if the results correlated to the high numbers of patients with COVID-19. Yet, current data did not show VAP improvement with reduced numbers of patients with COVID-19 admitted to the ICU. As a result, a motion was made by the committee recommending the creation of a special subcommittee to review and address concerns surrounding VAP. An interprofessional subcommittee immediately started meeting weekly in July. The subcommittee began with the purpose of reviewing the past several quarters/months of VAP data along with reviewing and revising critical care policies related to ventilator care or VAP. This interprofessional team included medical staff, nursing, clinical pharmacists, respiratory therapists, infection prevention, and quality.

PLANNING

The first step was to review the organization's policy compared with current evidence-based practices. During the review process, literature on evidence-based practice showed that a ventilator bundle approach should be implemented to standardize care and reduce infections. The goal of ventilator bundled care was aimed at preventing VAP, although there is little current evidence that supports the reduction of VAEs. The ventilator bundle is considered standardized care, and many times differ from varying organizations. Nonetheless, there are some core measures that are commonly seen. These core measures/practices include patient positioning, limiting the length of time on mechanical ventilation, interruption in sedation to determine spontaneous breathing, oral care, deep vein thrombosis (DVT) prophylaxis, stress ulcer prophylaxis, suctioning, and ventilator circuit care.[5]

One of the first and most common elements of bundled care is elevating the head of bed (HOB). A ventilated patient kept flat, and supine is a risk factor for developing pneumonia. Therefore, one of the simplest and least expensive tasks in VAP prevention bundled care is keeping the ventilated patient in a semirecumbent position. Studies have shown that having the HOB elevated 45° greatly reduced the rate of pneumonia in ventilated patients.[6] Although there is no clear evidence as to what degree the HOB should be elevated, the goal is to avoid lowing the HOB less than 30° unless there are other medical reasons to contraindicate the elevation.[7]

Another component of ventilator bundled care is avoiding or limiting the length of time on mechanical ventilation. Minimizing or reducing the amount of time a patient is subjected to mechanical ventilation is an extremely important practice to prevent VAP. Using other noninvasive approaches for airway maintenance are options to implement before or as an alternative if appropriate. Protocols such as ventilator weaning programs assist the team in evaluating the need for ventilation and progression to remove or modify the treatment.[8] Evidence also recommends performing spontaneous awakening trial (SAT) and spontaneous breathing trial (SBT) daily by pausing sedation to determine readiness for less ventilator support or to remove the ventilator. Trials have demonstrated that there is a decrease of 2 to 4 days of ventilator requirements when there is an interruption in sedation along with decreasing the overall sedation exposure. Sedation interruption allows the patient to be more awake to have better opportunity to pass the SBT.[9]

Oral care is also a strategy included as part of bundled care. There have been many studies and published articles on conducting oral care for ventilated patients. In a meta-analysis regarding the use of chlorhexidine oral care, the conclusion states there is statistically significant evidence that ventilated patients who receive oral care with chlorhexidine have a reduced risk of developing VAP.[10] Additionally, a Cochrane systematic review writes that chlorhexidine probably reduces VAP as the evidence indicates, with moderate certainty.[11,12] Last of all regarding oral hygiene, it is vital to perform oral care appropriately in the oral cavity. For the best results in preventing VAP, the treatment should start the same day as intubation, performed 4 times daily and continued until extubated.[13]

Other measures to reduce VAP are related to suctioning and ventilator circuit care. To prevent potential contamination, the recommendation is to reduce the frequency of times the ventilator circuit is broken by not disconnecting tubing and increasing the amount of time between circuit changes. No longer is it advised to change ventilator circuits daily but to increase the time between changes to 48 hours or longer. Along with keeping the circuits closed, using a closed suction catheter system also reduces the potential for contamination.[5,14]

Two other measures seem in the literature as part of the VAP prevention bundle that include prophylaxis for both DVT and stress ulcers. Conversely, there is no direct correlation between the prophylaxis measures and VAP. Critically ill patients are prone to both conditions, and therefore, it has been included in bundled care. Even though prevention of DVT and stress ulcers for ventilated patients are not necessarily related to VAP reduction, these interventions may reduce overall morbidity and mortality.[5]

The ICUs were already participating in the hospital's decolonization program. This program includes the use of chlorhexidine gluconate bathing and an alcohol-based product applied nasally. Decolonization has been identified as one intervention to decrease hospital-acquired infections.[15] During the initial subcommittee's meetings, the hospital infection control preventionist presented a recommendation requesting a review and consideration to change from the current nasal alcohol-based product to mupirocin in the ICUs. The use of mupirocin was found to be the most effective in eradicating methicillin-resistant *Staphylococcus aureus* (MRSA) with short-term usage of 4 to 7 days.[16] Consequently, the recommendation was accepted by the subcommittee to begin a pilot with mupirocin.

The current facility's policy and practice regarding ventilator care and VAP prevention was compared with current evidence-based practices regarding VAP bundled care in the literature. Similar care in the ventilator policy included elevating the HOB between 30° and 45°, SAT, SBT, along with deep venous thrombosis (DVT) prophylaxis measures. A critical care guideline provided an algorithm giving directions for nurses to conduct the SAT and respiratory therapy to conduct the SBT. Other bundled care measures such as closed suctioning system, circuit changes, hand hygiene, gloves, and turning were included in other departmental and hospital policies. A difference was noted regarding current practice related to oral care currently performed every 2 hours verses the recommended every 4 hours in the literature. The only bundled strategy not included in policies or guidelines was stress ulcer prophylaxis. **Table 1** outlines the ICU's practice compared with the literature regarding bundled care for VAP. The interprofessional subcommittee concluded that various interventions currently in practice were in line with the evidence-based VAP bundle. Recommended changes to current policies included having a VAP bundled care policy, changing oral care from every 2 hours to every 4 hours, and converting the alcohol-based nasal product to mupirocin in the decolonization policy. The current practice was for nursing and respiratory to alternate the oral care treatment. With this modification, the respiratory therapist would assume responsibility for all oral care every 4 hours with the goal of improving compliance.

Table 1
ICU's practice compared to the literature

Practice	VAP Bundle in Literature	Hospital Practice	Key
Head of Bed Elevated	30–45°	>30 degree	✔
Oral Care	Chlorhexidine every 4 h	Every 2 hours*	◆
Spontaneous Awakening Trial (SAT)	Daily	Yes, daily	✔
Spontaneous Breathing Trial (SBT)	Daily	Yes, daily	✔
Circuit Care	Reduce breaks in circuits	Other policy	✔
Suctioning	Closed	Yes, closed	✔
Deep Vein Thrombosis (DVT) prophylaxis	Included in bundle	Yes	✔
Stress ulcer prophylaxis	Included in bundle	No**	X
Hand Hygiene	Included in bundle	Other policy	✔
Turning	Included in bundle	Other policy	✔

Key: ✔: Performing standard. ◆: Not performing to standard. X: Not performing.

The subcommittee determined 2 modifications to practice were needed to implement the VAP bundle. The first recommendation would be to change from the current alcohol-based nasal product to mupirocin. The second suggestion included modifying oral care from every 2 hours to every 4 hours. Both proposals were presented to the critical care committee in September 2022 and approved with a goal of implementing the transformations in October 2022.

IMPLEMENTATION

The first hurdle was the conversion of the current nasal alcohol-based product to mupirocin. A request was made to the hospital's system information technology (IT) department to have mupirocin added to the ICU admission order set for a pilot. The request was denied because all the system hospitals use the same critical care order set and other hospitals in the system were not using mupirocin. Order sets only received approval for items that all hospitals in the system agreed on. To arrange for the mupirocin order to be added manually for admitted patients, the subcommittee partnered with clinical pharmacists who agreed to input the mupirocin order in the electronic medical record (EMR) when patients were admitted or transferred to one of the ICUs.

The quality nurse partnered with IT and developed an audit tool to review compliance with the VAP bundle. There was already an electronic report regarding the compliance rates for the decolonization program. This study entailed using the EMR and developing a report to determine if bundle elements were documented within the previous 24 hours. Once the report was generated from the EMR, it was able to capture HOB elevation, oral hygiene, and ventilator days. The report was validated by critical care nurse leaders while attending daily rounds with the Medical Director, Nursing Director, charge nurse, case management, physical therapy, dietary, and the bedside nurses. During rounds, the ventilator bundle was openly discussed while the EMR was open to review documentation. The VAP bundle compliance report was compared with actual documentation in the EMR during rounds. After a few minor adjustments, the electronic VAP bundle compliance report was deemed effective and reliable. **Table 2** shows a sample of the electronic VAP bundle compliance report. The electronic VAP bundle compliance report incorporates current compliance at the exact time of running the report. The electronic report is automatically e-mailed every morning to both the MICU and TICU nursing directors. Others, including the charge nurse can run the report ad hoc to look at compliance at any given time.

During rounds with nurses and respiratory therapists before implementing changes, the staff nurses and respiratory therapists were aware of VAP interventions and stated that care was being performed according to the policy. Yet, when performing preliminary audits, the compliance rate among both nurses and respiratory therapy staff was inconsistent regarding oral care every 2 hours according to the policy. Consequently, it was determined that all staff needed additional education on VAP, bundle care, and changes that were recently approved to the policy. Education was provided to all staff including nurses, respiratory therapists, and clinical pharmacists during individual departmental staff meetings regarding VAP, the new VAP bundle policy, and the responsibilities of each discipline. Nursing was educated on HOB, changes in oral care to every 4 hours performed by respiratory therapists, in addition to education regarding change in practice from current alcohol-based nasal product to mupirocin through online learning modules and a flyer (**Fig. 1**). Respiratory therapy was educated on modifications to oral hygiene changed to every 4 hours, only performed by a respiratory therapist. This change in practice regarding oral care incurred no change for respiratory but nursing would no longer be

Table 2			
Sample of electronic ventilator-associated pneumonia bundle compliance report			
MICU Bed	**HOB**	**Oral Care**	**Vent Days**
Bed 1	0	0	1
Bed 2	1	1	1
Bed 3	0	0	1
Bed 4	0	0	2
Bed 5	0	0	2
Bed 6	1	1	3
Bed 7	1	1	3
Bed 8	0	0	4
Bed 9	0	1	5
Bed 10	1	0	5
Bed 11	0	1	6
Bed 12	0	0	6
Bed 13	0	0	6
Bed 14	1	0	6
Bed 15	1	1	6
MICU Total	40%	40%	57
TICU Bed	**HOB**	**Oral Care**	**Vent Days**
Bed 1	1	1	1
Bed 2	0	1	1
Bed 3	0	1	5
Bed 4	0	1	6
Bed 5	1	1	6
Bed 6	1	1	6
Bed 7	0	0	6
Bed 8	1	0	6
Bed 9	0	1	6
Bed 10	1	0	6
Bed 11	1	1	6
Bed 12	0	0	6
Bed 13	1	1	6
Bed 14	0	1	6
Bed 15	0	0	6
Bed 16	1	0	6
TICU Total	50%	63%	85

0, noncompliant with intervention; 1, compliant with intervention.

performing oral care in between respiratory therapists' treatments. The clinical pharmacists were involved with the subcommittee and were aware of the need to input an order for mupirocin.

OUTCOMES

Full implementation of the revised VAP bundle policy, converting to mupirocin along with monitoring the electronic compliance reports for both decolonization and VAP

What is it?

- Mupirocin is a topical antibiotic that can be used to decolonize or eradicate MRSA and MSSA from patient's nares. This helps prevent more severe infections like central line associated blood stream infection and bacteremia.

Why are we piloting mupirocin?

- ICUs continues to have hospital onset (HO) MRSA bacteremia at a higher rate than expected when compared to other like hospitals.
- Decolonization, including nasal mupirocin and CHG bathing, has been shown to reduce 37% of clinical MRSA cultures and 44% of all-cause bloodstream infections.

How long will we be piloting mupirocin?

- Our plan is to begin on October 3 and pilot Mupirocin for 3 months after which a small group will review our infection data. If there's sufficient data, we will determine whether to continue the pilot as a permanent workflow or revert back to using the Nozin decolonization product.

How will the mupirocin order be placed?

- The Critical Care PharmD will convert orders from Nozin to Mupirocin Monday thru Friday on all ICU patients admitted. On weekends, the ICU Charge nurse will notify pharmacy to update orders on any patients without mupirocin ordered.

How often is mupirocin applied?

- Mupirocin should be administered to patients admitted to MICU, and TICU twice a day for 5 days, starting on day 1 of admission.
- The protocol will stop upon discharge or transfer from critical care.
- The protocol will restart from the beginning for patients readmitted to critical care, regardless of the duration of absence.

Do we still have to give Nozin to patients during the trial?

- No, we will not be administering Nozin to patients on MICU, and TICU during the trial. All supply of Nozin will be removed from the unit and only mupirocin will be administered to patients.
- Patients on non-critical care units will continue to use Nozin for nasal decolonization.

How to apply nasal mupirocin:

- Have patient blow their nose to empty their nostrils.
- Place patient's bed at 30 degrees, if tolerated.
- Apply 0.5 g (pea-sized) amount of mupirocin onto sterile cotton swab.
- Apply swab directly into nostril.
- Repeat for other nostril.
- Press nostrils together and massage gently for 60 seconds.
- Do this twice a day for 5 days during ICU stay.
- Avoid contact with eyes and other intranasal products.
- If nasal devices are in place (e.g., nasal intubation, NG tubes), place mupirocin around tubing and massage gently to distribute ointment.
- If 2 or more doses are missed, re-start the protocol.

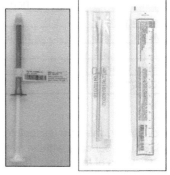

Fig. 1. Mupirocin nasal decolonization pilot.

bundle usage, started on October 1, 2022. At the end of the first quarter, VAP bundle compliance was 90.62% for HOB elevation and 93.32% for oral care. Compliance with VAP bundle care demonstrated more improvement in the first quarter of 2023 with HOB 96% and 94.56% for oral care (**Table 3**). The VAP and VAE rates increased during the third quarter of 2022, at which time the subcommittee was meeting and planning. Nevertheless, the fourth quarter of 2022 showed improvement during previous quarters. In the first quarter of 2023, the VAP rate did not continue to demonstrate significant improvement. The VAE rates on the other hand continued to show improvement (**Fig. 2**).

Gains can continue to occur with persistent improvements in compliance and continuous education for staff.[17] With every VAP reduction, there is potential for cost avoidance or cost savings to the facility. According to the Agency for Research

Table 3
Bundled compliance rates

	2022 4th Quarter		
	Bundle Compliance Rates		
Date	Unit	HOB	Oral Care
October	MICU	85.32%	93.32%
	TICU	97.37%	92.37%
October Total		91.34%	92.84%
November	MICU	81.94%	91.89%
	TICU	92.94%	93.76%
November Total		87.29%	92.80%
December	MICU	89.75%	97.45%
	TICU	95.95%	91.00%
December Total		92.85%	94.23%
2022 Q4 Total		90.62%	94.23%
	2023 1st Quarter		
	Bundle Compliance Rates		
Date	Unit	HOB	Oral Care
January	MICU	97.53%	96.91%
	TICU	92.00%	96.00%
January Total		95.78%	96.62%
February	MICU	96.30%	88.89%
	TICU	95.77%	88.73%
February Total		96.05%	88.82%
March	MICU	94.95%	97.50%
	TICU	98.00%	99.00%
March Total		96.48%	98.25%
2023 Q1 Total		99.00%	94.56%

and Quality, the cost associated with a VAP diagnosis range from US$19,325 to US$80,013 per case with an average cost of US$47,238.[18] This project had an actual cost savings of more than US$21,000 by converting the oral hygiene kits from every 2 hours to every 4 hours.

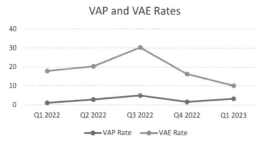

Fig. 2. Critical care VAP and VAE rates.

SUMMARY

Providing consistent evidence based bundled care for critically ill patients on a ventilator has been proven to reduce VAP. Preventing these HACs will reduce the amount of time spent in the ICU as well as overall length of stay for patients in the hospital. More importantly, implementation of VAP bundles can reduce overall morbidity and mortality.[19] Although this quality improvement project is still in the early implementation stage, there are additional opportunities for improvement in monitoring compliance including expanding the electronic VAP bundle compliance report to include SAT and SBT documentation in the EMR. The critical care committee should also consider adding stress ulcer prophylaxis to the VAP bundle with implementation in the third quarter of 2023.

CLINICS CARE POINTS

- Interprofessional team work aimed in standardizing bundle compliance can improve VAP.
- Consistency in applying standard care is key.
- Comparing and contrasting evidence based practices to current practice is the first step.
- Having electronic audits and monitoring for leaders and staff makes reviewing the standard dialy less burdensome.

REFERENCES

1. AHRQ Tools To Reduce Hospital-Acquired Conditions. Agency for Healthcare Research and Quality Web site. Available: https://www.ahrq.gov/hai/hac/tools.html. Published December 2016. Updated February 2023. Accessed May 5, 2023.
2. Buterakos R, Jenkins P, Cranford J, et al. An in-dept look at ventilator-associated pneumonia in trauma patients and efforts to increase bundle compliance, education, and documentation in a surgical trauma critical care unit. Am J Infect Control 2022;50:1333–8.
3. Ventilator-Associated Event (VAE). Centers for Disease Control and Prevention Web site. Available: https://www.cdc.gov/nhsn/pdfs/pscmanual/10-vae_final.pdf Published January 2023. Assessed May 5, 2023.
4. Isac C, Prevention of VAP John A. Endless evolving evidence-systematic literature review. Nurs Forum 2021;56:905–15.
5. Kallet R. Ventilator bundles in transition: from prevention of ventilator-associated pneumonia to prevention of ventilator-associated events. Respir Care 2019;64(8):994–1006.
6. Drakulovic M, Torres A, Bauer T, et al. Supine body position as a risk factor for nosocomial pneumonia in mechanically ventilated patients: a randomized trial. Lancet 1999;354:1851–8.
7. Guner C. Role of head-of-bed elevation in preventing ventilator-associated pneumonia bed elevation and pneumonia. Nurs Crit Care 2022;27:635–45.
8. Boltey E, Yakusheva O, Costa D. 5 Nursing strategies to prevent ventilator-associated pneumonia. Am Nurse Today 2017;12(6):42–3.
9. Klompas M, Branson R, Eichenwald E, et al. Strategies to prevent ventilator-associated pneumonia in acute care hospitals: 2014 update. Infect Control Hosp Epidemiol 2014;35(8):915–36.

10. Dia W, Lin Y, Yang X, et al. Meta-analysis of the efficacy and safety of chlorhexidine for ventilator-associate pneumonia prevention in mechanically ventilated patients. Evid base Compl Alternative Med 2022. https://doi.org/10.1155/2022/5311034.
11. Shi Z, Xie H, Wang P, et al. Oral hygiene care for critically ill patients to prevent ventilator-associated pneumonia (Review). Cochrane Database Syst Rev 2013. https://doi.org/10.1002/14651858.CD008367.pub2.
12. Cooper A. Oral hygiene care to prevent ventilator-associated pneumonia in critically ill patients. Crit Care Nurse 2021;41(4):80–3.
13. Zuckerman L. Oral chlorhexidine use to prevent ventilator-associated pneumonia in adults. Dimens Crit Care Nurs 2016;35(1):25–36.
14. Sanie S, Rahnemayan S, Javan S, et al. Comparison of closed vs open suction in prevention of ventilator-associated pneumonia: a systematic review and meta-analysis. Indian J Crit Care Med 2022;26(7):839–45.
15. Pratt N, Heishman C, Blizard K, et al. Alcohol-based nasal decolonization and chlorhexidine bathing to reduce methicillin-resistant staphylococcus aureus hospital-acquired infections in critical patients. Am J Infect Control 2022;50(2022):31.
16. Ammeriaan H, Kluytmans J, Wertheim H, et al. Eradication of methicillin-resistant staphylococcus aureus carriage: a systematic review. Healthcare Epidemiology 2009;48:922–30.
17. Rello J, Afonso E, Lisba T, et al. A care approach for prevention of ventilator-associated pneumonia. Clin Microbiol Infect 2012;19:363–9.
18. AHRQ Estimating the Additional Hospital Inpatient cost and Mortality Associated with Selected Hospital Acquired Conditions:Agency for Healthcare Research and Quality Web site. Available at: https://www.ahrq.gov/hai/pfp/haccost2017-results.html. Published November 2017. Accessed May 23, 2023.
19. Ladbrook E, Khaw D, Bouchoucha S, et al. A systematic scoping review of the cost-impact of ventilator-associated pneumonia (VAP) intervention bundles in intensive care. Am J Infect Control 2021;49(2021):928–36.

Polypharmacy in the Cardiovascular Geriatric Critical Care Population
Improving Outcomes

Chloé Davidson Villavaso, MN, APRN, ACNS-BC, CV-BC, CMC, FPCNA, AACC[a],*,
Shavonne Williams, MN, APRN, ACNS-BC, ANVP-BC, SCRN, CCRN-K[b,1],
Tracy M. Parker, MSN, APRN, FNP-BC[c]

KEYWORDS

- Polypharmacy • Critical care • Cardiovascular • Geriatric • Deprescribing
- Team-based care

KEY POINTS

- Polypharmacy increases the risk of adverse outcomes in the cardiovascular geriatric critical care population.
- Age-related physiologic changes, the critical care environment, and polypharmacy heighten the complexity of the cardiovascular geriatric critical care population.
- Tools to assist with appropriate prescribing and deprescribing are available and can be used by the interprofessional team.

INTRODUCTION

Aging is a complex transition comprised of physiologic and cognitive changes. The cardiovascular geriatric population requiring intensive or critical care is a group vulnerable to adverse outcomes as a result of age, the critical care environment, geriatric syndromes, and multiple chronic conditions. Polypharmacy is a common diagnosis in this population as a result of comorbid conditions. Due to the projected increase in polypharmacy in the cardiovascular geriatric critical care population (CGCP), interventions to improve care in this group will be discussed.

[a] Clinical Faculty, Tulane University School of Medicine, Heart and Vascular Institute, 1430 Tulane Avenue #8548, New Orleans, LA 70112, USA; [b] Texas Health Presbyterian Hospital, Dallas, TX, USA; [c] Touro Heart and Vascular Care, LCMC Health, 3715 Prytania Street, Suite 400, New Orleans, LA 70115, USA
[1] Present address: 3540 East Broad Street Suite 120-226, Mansfield, TX 76063.
* Corresponding author.
E-mail address: cvillavaso@tulane.edu

Crit Care Nurs Clin N Am 35 (2023) 505–512
https://doi.org/10.1016/j.cnc.2023.05.012
0899-5885/23/© 2023 Elsevier Inc. All rights reserved.
ccnursing.theclinics.com

STATE OF THE ISSUE

The geriatric population, age 65 and over, is the fastest growing sector of the United States population and makes up a significant proportion of persons with cardiovascular disease (CVD).[1] Over 60% of patients with CVD are over age 69. Additionally, more than 85% are over 85 years of age.[2] While critical care units are designed to address acute, high-acuity conditions, the environment can adversely affect the geriatric population. For example, critical care environments expose patients to bed rest, sedation, sensory stressors, new medications, disorientation, and disruptions in sleep, dietary, and excretion routines.[2] Furthermore, the components of geriatric syndrome, frailty, delirium, multimorbidity, immobility, malnutrition, and end-of-life and palliative care needs, further complicate the care required by the older adult population.[2]

Geriatric adults face age-related changes adding to the complexity of caring for this group of patients. Physiologic cardiovascular changes in the geriatric population include vascular stiffening, reduction in the number of myocytes and sinus node cells, and remodeling of the left ventricle.[3] Such changes can lead to decreased contractility, myocardial compliance, and beta adrenergic sensitivity, and increased ventricular filling pressures.[3] **Table 1** lists age-related cardiovascular changes and potential clinical associations. In addition, reduced renal function and hepatic clearance and greater percentage of body fat effect drug pharmacokinetics and pharmacodynamics in older adults.[2]

Due to the multimorbid conditions present in the cardiovascular geriatric population, numerous medications are frequently prescribed. Commonly prescribed cardiovascular medications include antihypertensives, diuretics, antiplatelets, anticoagulants, electrolyte supplements, lipid-lowering medications, nitrates, antiarrhythmics, and inotropic and chronotropic agents.[4]

POLYPHARMACY

The word polypharmacy is used widely in medical literature; however, there is no consensual definition. Polypharmacy has been described as the use of multiple medications concurrently, medication duplication, and potentially inappropriate drug use.[5] For the purpose of this article, polypharmacy is defined as five or more medications used concurrently, including over-the-counter medications.[6]

The prevalence of polypharmacy in the geriatric population rose from 24% to 39% from 2000 to 2012.[7] Furthermore, polypharmacy is known to increase the risk of adverse drug events, falls, drug-drug interactions, noncompliance, financial burden, and geriatric syndromes.[1] In addition to commonly prescribed cardiovascular medications, other prescribed and over-the-counter medications are frequently included such as analgesics, laxatives, antacids, antibiotics, herbal supplements, cough and cold medications, and vitamins and minerals. In a study aiming to address the knowledge gap related to harm associated with polypharmacy in patients with heart failure,

Table 1	
Age-related cardiovascular changes and clinical associations	
Age-Related Cardiovascular Changes	**Clinical Associations**
• Vascular stiffening	• Systolic hypertension
• Decreased number of myocytes	• Left ventricular dysfunction
• Left ventricular remodeling	• Valvular disfunction
• Reduced number of sinus node cells	• Heart failure with preserved ejection fraction
• Decreased nitrous oxide production	• Pulmonary hypertension
• Increased valvular calcium	

investigators noted participants were on more noncardiac medications compared to heart failure and nonheart failure cardiovascular medications.[4] This further supports the need for interventions to address polypharmacy.

DEPRESCRIBING

Deprescribing is the practice of decreasing the number of medications taken and/or decreasing the dose. Deprescribing is carried out in a systematic method which includes identifying medications that cause potential harm while considering the patient's treatment goals.[8] Although deprescribing has been shown to safely reduce the number of potentially harmful medications, falls, change in mental status, emergency room visits, and major complications, literature demonstrating a decrease in mortality, hospitalization, and an improvement in quality of life is lacking.[8–10]

Several barriers to deprescribing have been documented. Investigators of a qualitative study exploring physicians' knowledge and barriers to deprescribing reported the lack of knowledge regarding the process of deprescribing, fear of conflict with clinical pharmacists, lack of coordination of care, time constraints, and patient resistance as barriers to deprescribing.[11] The lack of organizational culture supporting deprescribing is an additional challenge to consider.[12] Goyal and colleagues[13] evaluated clinicians' perspectives toward deprescribing finding cardiologists least likely to deprescribe cardiovascular medications in patients with limited life expectancy and when adverse drug events occurred. This finding highlights the need for evidence-based interventions to address polypharmacy in the CGCP.

TOOLS TO FACILITATE APPROPRIATE PRESCRIBING AND APPROPRIATE DEPRESCRIBING

Several validated tools are available to guide clinicians in appropriately prescribing and deprescribing medications (**Box 1**). These tools can be applied to the CGCP. In 2019, the American Geriatric Society Beers Criteria was updated.[14] This compilation of medications classifies drugs into categories that should be avoided in most older adults based on the individual safety risk. The Beers Criteria recommends healthcare providers should consider patient diagnoses, medications with a high likelihood of drug-drug interactions, those posing a high risk for harmful side effects, and medications which should be avoided or dosed specifically for renal impairment.[8,14]

The Medication Appropriateness Index (MAI) consists of 10 questions related to the indication, effectiveness, dosage, instructions, interactions, duplication, and duration of drug therapy.[15] Each question is assigned a weighted score between 1 and 3. The resulting score ranges from zero, indicating the medication is most appropriate, to 18, indicating the medication is least appropriate.[15]

Box 1
Applicable CGCP tools

Prescribing and Deprescribing Tools
- Beers Criteria
- Medication Appropriateness Index (MAI)
- CEASE algorithm
- Deprescribing Protocol
- Good Palliative-Geriatric Practice algorithm
- Screening Tool of Older People's Prescriptions (STOPP)
- Screening Tool to Alert Doctors to the Right Treatment (START)

Another deprescribing tool mentioned in the literature is the CEASE algorithm. This process addresses the Current medications, Elevated risk of the medication, Assessing the usefulness of the medication, Sorting medications for discontinuation by identifying those with the lowest benefit and ease of discontinuation, and Eliminating medications using a discontinuation regimen and monitoring the patient's outcomes.[16]

The Deprescribing Protocol proposed by Scott and colleagues[17] is comprised of the following steps:

1. Obtaining a list of the patient's current medications
2. Considering the risks of harmful medication effects
3. Evaluating each medication for discontinuation eligibility
4. First, discontinuing medications with the greatest possible harm. Second, discontinuing those with the lowest risk of withdrawal and negative effects. Third, discontinuing medications the patient is most in favor of eliminating.
5. Educating the patient on the medication plan and monitor for untoward reactions (**Fig. 1**).

The Good Palliative-Geriatric Practice algorithm uses a series of questions to facilitate collaboration between the patient, the support system, and clinician to discontinue medications lacking lifesaving benefit. The Good Palliative-Geriatric Practice algorithm focuses on the patient characteristics of advanced age, comorbid conditions, frailty, dementia, and limited life expectancy as the framework for deprescribing.[18]

Additional deprescribing tools highlighted in the literature include the Screening Tool of Older People's Prescriptions (STOPP) and the Screening Tool to Alert Doctors to the Right Treatment (START) which aid in medication appropriateness by advising on inappropriate and undersprescribed medications.[8] Furthermore, the Drug Burden Index identifies the burden of anticholinergic and sedative medications.[8] Lastly, the Anticholinergic Risk Scale and the Anticholinergic Drug Scale characterize the burden and risk of adverse drug events associated with anticholinergic use.[8]

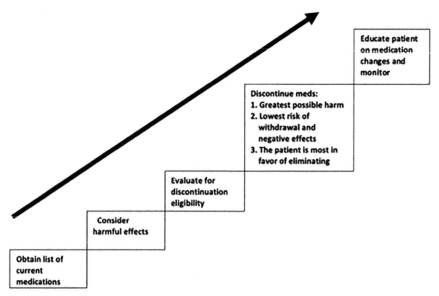

Fig. 1. Deprescribing steps.

TEAM-BASED APPROACH TO POLYPHARMACY

Team-based care is defined as two or more healthcare members collaborating with the patient and the patient's support system to achieve shared goals, coordinate care, and improve outcomes.[19] Given the complexity of decision-making required to deliver appropriate care to older adults in the cardiac intensive care unit, The American Heart Association released a scientific statement supporting the use of interprofessional team-based care.[2]

Members of the interprofessional team include the patient and the patient's personal support system, critical care clinical nurse specialists, clinical pharmacists, nurse practitioners, physician assistants, physicians, critical care registered nurses, allied health professionals, and social workers.[20–23] **Fig. 2** displays a conceptual model of a team-based approach to addressing polypharmacy. With the patient at the center of the interprofessional team, continuous collaboration occurs between healthcare team members, while shared decision-making occurs between the patient and the prescribing team members. Shared decision-making is the process of merging the patient's preferences and goals for treatment with evidence-based practice to provide individualized care.[2] The literature supports implementing shared-decision making via an interprofessional approach.[24] To successfully facilitate shared decision-making, it is the responsibility of the healthcare team to establish trust with the patient and their support system.

ROLES OF THE INTERPROFESSIONAL TEAM

Each member of the interprofessional team brings a unique knowledge base and perspective to the care of the CGCP. Although there is the possibility of role overlap, members may assume roles more frequently based on education and training. The following is a proposed description of the roles of the interprofessional team members.

The patient and support system-integrate information and recommendations from the interprofessional team with personal preferences and social determinants to select treatment. The clinical pharmacists evaluate for polypharmacy, identifies medications eligible for discontinuation, and makes recommendations for deprescribing.[25,26] The prescribing members of the interprofessional team are the physicians, critical care clinical nurse specialists, nurse practitioners, and physician assistants. Since the

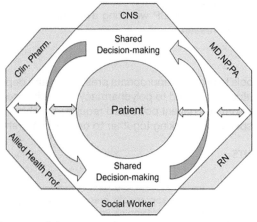

Fig. 2. Team-based care model.

role of the clinical nurse specialist may vary depending on practice location, the role will be described separately from the other prescribing clinicians.

The critical care clinical nurse specialist may lead the interprofessional team efforts to address polypharmacy through team education, facilitating effective team communication, identify gaps in care, recommending and critically evaluating evidence-based practice change to improve outcomes, and leading quality improvement efforts.[20,27,28] The physicians, nurse practitioners, and physician assistants contribute to the team by continuously evaluating the patient's medication list, considering recommendations for deprescribing from the clinical pharmacists and other members of the team, prioritizing medications eligible for discontinuation, leading the collaborative discussion with the patient regarding the treatment plan, and ordering the deprescribing monitoring protocol.[21,24,29,30] The critical care registered nurses collaborate with the team to report changes in the patient's clinical status with a focus on drug-drug interactions, prescribing cascades, adverse reactions, communicating discrepancies in medication reconciliation, and carrying out deprescribing and monitoring protocols.[31,32] Social workers are vital to address social determinants of health which facilitates continuity of care during care transitions.

Although several deprescribing tools exist, the clinical members of the interprofessional team should decide which tool or tools to implement. In addition to the stated interventions, the interprofessional team can incorporate the electronic health record (EHR) into efforts to address polypharmacy by ensuring the patient's medications are linked to a diagnosis and transferred to subsequent levels of care, including discharge. Members of the interprofessional team can attend daily patient rounds to ensure coordination and continuity of care. Prescribing clinicians should remain attentive to prescribing alerts to avoid drug-drug interactions, inappropriate prescribing, and incorporate deprescribing.

RECOMMENDATIONS FOR FUTURE RESEARCH

Future research is needed to strengthen the evidence to support interventions aimed at improving the care of the CGCP. Additional research is needed regarding whether deprescribing improves outcomes and quality of care and reduces adverse events in older adults with acute cardiovascular conditions. Further research on the effects of clinician-led deprescribing interventions will support evidence-based care in the CGCP. In addition, studies focused on the effects of drugs on older adults will aid in reducing medication-associated adverse events.[2] Studies emphasizing the prevalence of polypharmacy in the CGCP will bring awareness to the scope of the issue and likely prompt future research.

SUMMARY

Evidence-based tools to promote appropriate prescribing and deprescribing are available to improve outcomes related to polypharmacy in cardiovascular geriatric critical care patients. This complex patient populated requires a highly integrated team consisting of various specialties working together to deliver comprehensive care.

CLINICS CARE POINTS

- Evidence-based tools to facilitate appropriate prescribing and deprescribing include the Beers Criteria, Screening Tool of Older People's Prescriptions (STOPP), Screening Tool to Alert Doctors to the Right Treatment (START), Medication Appropriateness Index (MAI),

CEASE algorithm, Deprescribing Protocol, Good Palliative-Geriatric Practice algorithm, Drug Burden Index, and the Anticholinergic Risk Scale.

- An interprofessional critical care team implementing shared decision-making with the patient, evidence-based prescribing and deprescribing tools, and care coordination supports optimal outcomes for the cardiovascular geriatric critical care population.

DISCLOSURE

The authors have nothing to disclose.

ACKNOWLEDGMENTS

Branden Jude Villavaso, Jr.: **Fig. 2**.

REFERENCES

1. Shah BM, Hajjar ER. Polypharmacy, adverse drug reactions, and geriatric syndromes. Clin Geriatr Med 2012;28(2):173–86.
2. Damluji AA, Forman DE, van Diepen S, et al. Older adults in the cardiac intensive care Unit: factoring geriatric syndromes in the management, prognosis, and process of care: a scientific statement from the American heart association. Circulation 2020;141(2):e6–32.
3. Pauldine R. Geriatric cardiovascular critical care. In: Akhtar S, Rosenbaum S, editors. Principles pf geriatric critical care. Cambridge: Cambridge University Press; 2018. p. 81–101. https://doi.org/10.1017/9781316676325.007.
4. Unlu O, Levitan EB, Reshetnyak E, et al. Polypharmacy in older adults hospitalized for heart failure. Circulation Heart failure 2020;13(11):e006977.
5. Mortazavi SS, Shati M, Keshtkar A, et al. Defining polypharmacy in the elderly: a systematic review protocol. BMJ Open 2016;6(3):e010989.
6. World Health Organization. (2019). Safety in polypharmacy. Retrieved on April 20, 2023 Available at: https://www.who.int/docs/default-source/patient-safety/who-uhc-sds-2019-11-eng.pdf. Accessed April 20, 2023.
7. Kantor ED, Rehm CD, Haas JS, et al. Trends in prescription drug Use among adults in the United States from 1999-2012. JAMA, J Am Med Assoc 2015;314(17):1818–30.
8. Rochon PA, Petrovic M, Cherubini A, et al. Polypharmacy, inappropriate prescribing, and deprescribing in older people: through a sex and gender lens. The Lancet Healthy longevity 2021;2(5):e290–300.
9. Pruskowski JA, Springer S, Thorpe CT, et al. Does deprescribing improve quality of life? A systematic review of the literature. Drugs Aging 2019;36(12):1097–110.
10. Garfinkel D. Poly-de-prescribing to treat polypharmacy: efficacy and safety. Therapeutic advances in drug safety 2018;9(1):25–43.
11. AlRasheed MM, Alhawassi TM, Alanazi A, et al. Knowledge and willingness of physicians about deprescribing among older patients: a qualitative study. Clin Interv Aging 2018;13:1401–8.
12. Conklin J, Farrell B, Suleman S. Implementing deprescribing guidelines into frontline practice: barriers and facilitators. Res Soc Adm Pharm 2019;15(6):796–800.
13. Goyal P, Anderson TS, Bernacki GM, et al. Physician perspectives on deprescribing cardiovascular medications for older adults. J Am Geriatr Soc 2020;68(1):78–86.

14. Kurczewska-Michalak M, Lewek P, Jankowska-Polańska B, et al. Polypharmacy management in the older adults: a scoping review of available interventions. Front Pharmacol 2021;12:734045.

15. Hanlon JT, Schmader KE, Samsa GP, et al. A method for assessing drug therapy appropriateness. Journal of clinical epidemiology 1992;45(10):1045–51.

16. Scott IA, Le Couteur DG. Physicians need to take the lead in deprescribing. Intern Med J 2015;45(3):352–6.

17. Scott IA, Hilmer SN, Reeve E, et al. Reducing inappropriate polypharmacy: the process of deprescribing. JAMA Intern Med 2015;175(5):827–34.

18. Garfinkel D, Zur-Gil S, Ben-Israel J. The war against polypharmacy: a new cost-effective geriatric-palliative approach for improving drug therapy in disabled elderly people. Isr Med Assoc J 2007;9(6):430–4.

19. Smith CD, Balatbat C, Corbridge S, et al. Implementing optimal team-based care to reduce clinician burnout. NAM Perspectives 2018;8(9).

20. Gabbard ER, Klein D, Vollman K, et al. Clinical nurse specialist: a critical member of the ICU team. Clin Nurse Spec 2021;35(5):271–6.

21. Mangin D, Lamarche L, Agarwal G, et al. Team approach to polypharmacy evaluation and reduction: study protocol for a randomized controlled trial. Curr Contr Trials Cardiovasc Med 2021;22(1):746.

22. Muhandiramge J, Dev T, Kong J, et al. In-hospital deprescribing in the real world – a clinician-led approach to hyperpolypharmacy. J Pharm Pract Res 2023. https://doi.org/10.1002/jppr.1844.

23. Dharmarajan TS, Choi H, Hossain N, et al. Deprescribing as a clinical improvement focus. J Am Med Dir Assoc 2020;21(3):355–60.

24. Michalsen A, Long AC, DeKeyser Ganz F, et al. Interprofessional shared decision-making in the ICU: a systematic review and recommendations from an expert panel. Crit Care Med 2019;47(9):1258–66.

25. Kimura T, Fujita M, Shimizu M, et al. Effectiveness of pharmacist intervention for deprescribing potentially inappropriate medications: a prospective observational study. Journal of pharmaceutical health care and sciences 2022;8(1):12.

26. Byrne A, Byrne S, Dalton K. A pharmacist's unique opportunity within a multidisciplinary team to reduce drug-related problems for older adults in an intermediate care setting. Res Soc Adm Pharm 2022;18(4):2625–33.

27. Avery LJ, Schnell-Hoehn KN. Clinical nurse specialist practice in evidence-informed multidisciplinary cardiac care. Clin Nurse Spec 2010;24(2):76–9.

28. Ng B, Duong M, Lo S, et al. Deprescribing perceptions and practice reported by multidisciplinary hospital clinicians after, and by medical students before and after, viewing an e-learning module. Res Soc Adm Pharm 2021;17(11):1997–2005.

29. Potter EL, Lew TE, Sooriyakumaran M, et al. Evaluation of pharmacist-led physician-supported inpatient deprescribing model in older patients admitted to an acute general medical unit. Australasian journal on ageing 2019;38(3):206–10.

30. Delara M, Murray L, Jafari B, et al. Prevalence and factors associated with polypharmacy: a systematic review and meta-analysis. BMC Geriatr 2022;22(1):601.

31. Cateau D, Ballabeni P, Niquille A. Effects of an interprofessional deprescribing intervention in Swiss nursing homes: the Individual Deprescribing Intervention (IDeI) randomised controlled trial. BMC Geriatr 2021;21(1):655.

32. Krishnaswami A, Steinman MA, Goyal P, et al. Deprescribing in older adults with cardiovascular disease. J Am Coll Cardiol 2019;73(20):2584–95.

Acute Care for Elders and Nurses Improving Care for Health System Elders Models in Acute Care

Are We Still Using These Geriatric Models of Care?

Quinn Lacey, PhD, RN, CCRN

KEYWORDS

• Patient-centered care models • Older adult • Quality of care • Costs

KEY POINTS

- The Acute Care for Elders Unit model of care.
- The Nurses Improving Care for Health System Elders program.
- Hospital-acquired disability.
- Geriatric resource nurse.

INTRODUCTION

Being hospitalized can increase patients' chances of harm simply by mere exposure to predictable hazards encountered in the hospital and not by improper medical care.[1] Older patients are at particular risk for functional and mental decline due to hospitalization. These risks are compounded when patients are admitted into the intensive care unit (ICU) due to the nature of critical care and often the patient's limited mobility.[2] Acute illness, as often seen in the ICU, also disrupts the lives of older adults who rely on familiarity and routine. Since the 1980s, there have been recommendations within the literature to investigate special-care units for the elderly that minimize hazards from hospitalizations for the elderly. This article will examine 2 particular models that were created to improve the quality of care and reduce functional disability of older adults during acute illness and hospitalization: The Acute Care for Elders (ACE) Unit model and The Nurses Improving Care for Health System Elders (NICHE) program, both developed during the last 3 decades. What have we learned, and are we still using these geriatric models of care?

School of Nursing, LSU Health-New Orleans, 1900 Gravier Street, New Orleans, LA 70112, USA
E-mail address: qlace1@lsuhsc.edu

Crit Care Nurs Clin N Am 35 (2023) 513–521
https://doi.org/10.1016/j.cnc.2023.05.010
0899-5885/23/© 2023 Elsevier Inc. All rights reserved.
ccnursing.theclinics.com

BACKGROUND

In 1999, the Institute of Medicine Report *To Err is Human* concluded that preventable errors in care were the cause of tens of thousands of deaths in America.[3] Before this landmark report, in the early 90s, forward-thinking geriatric clinicians sought to develop conceptual models for caring for older adults in critical care that would primarily prevent hospital-acquired disability. This was the beginning of what would become known as the quality movement in health care. The ACE Units and model of care were developed during this time. Before the ACE model, 1992 saw the creation of The NICHE program. The ACE model and the NICHE program sought to improve the quality of care for older adults in the hospital environment.

Hospital-Acquired Disability

Hospital-acquired disability is typically defined as a net loss in the ability to perform one of the basic activities of daily living (ADL) without assistance, such as bathing, using the toilet, rising from a chair or a bed, or walking across the room by discharge.[4] Several hospital-related factors have been identified within the literature to contribute to a hospital-acquired disability, including limited mobility while hospitalized, little encouragement for independence, and undernutrition.[5] There are also numerous anxiety-provoking situations older adults must face being hospitalized, not to mention those potential hazards they or their families may not have considered. Restriction of physical mobility and loss of independence can lead to hospital-acquired disability.[5]

Older adults admitted to the hospital usually come with chronic illnesses into an unfamiliar and often restrictive environment. Several geriatric syndromes resemble hospital-acquired disabilities. Due to the stress of acute illness on older adults, it is often difficult to differentiate geriatric syndromes such as falls, incontinence, and delirium from hospital-acquired disabilities.[5] Geriatric syndromes occur insidiously over time. With the accumulation of comorbidities such as geriatric syndromes, including cognitive impairment and depression, the acute stress and confinement of a new environment can potentiate hospital-acquired disability.[6]

Between 1994 and 2009, spending on postacute care, rehabilitation, and skilled nursing was the fastest-growing major spending category and accounted for a large portion of spending growth in the United States (US).[7] Postacute care services such as in-patient rehabilitation, rehabilitation through home health, and skilled-nursing facilities today cost the American taxpayer US$57 billion annually.[8] There are estimates that as many as 30% of all patients aged older than 70 years who were hospitalized due to a medical illness were discharged with a hospital-acquired disability that they were not admitted with.[9] As mentioned previously, there are many factors associated with hospital-acquired disability that are not modifiable such as age, comorbidities, and severity of illness causing hospitalization. Still, there are hospital-related factors that can be targeted. These hospital-related factors are the targets of the ACE model and the NICHE program. This article aims to answer the question: Are we still using these geriatric models of care, and are they helping curb an annual cost of US$57 billion in critical care?

The Acute Care for Elders Unit Model

The ACE model was launched at the University Hospitals of Cleveland under the leadership of Dr Robert Palmer and the late Dr Jerome Kowal during the 90s, with its first publication in the New England Journal of Medicine in 1995.[10] The 5 essential elements of the model were as follows.

1. A prepared environment
2. A patient-centered assessment
3. A medical care review
4. Daily rounds (w/interprofessional team)
5. Early planning for discharge

To capture the first of the 5 essential elements of the ACE model, the Cleveland group envisioned an ergonomically enhanced environment for hospitalized geriatric patients. This included carpeted floors, dresser drawers for self-care items to assist with reorientation, and replacing the sterile feel of a hospital with a more home-like feel. Next, a patient-centered assessment was to be achieved by an interdisciplinary team that would round daily, centering on ADL, continence, early ambulation, and nutrition; a medical care review by a geriatrician/or geriatric pharmacist would monitor any medications with untoward effects on the older adult such as anticholinergics and monitor for unnecessary tethers such as Foleys and oxygen tubing. Early discharge planning was the fifth and final essential element of the original ACE model.[10]

Benefits published in the original randomized controlled trial (RCT) by the Cleveland group in 1995 comparing the ACE model to "usual care" concluded improvement in performing ADLs, shorter length of stay (LOS), lower hospital costs, and fewer discharges to institutions within the experimental group. The goal was to discharge the patient at their prehospital level of ADLs.[11] The original RCT in 1995 was performed at the University Hospitals of Cleveland in a university setting. A subsequent RCT by Counsel and colleagues[12] using 1531 patients aged older than 70 years in a community hospital found differences in ADL decline between the intervention group and the group receiving usual care. Fewer in the intervention group experienced a decline in ADLs or nursing home placement (34% vs 40%, respectively; P = .027). The researchers also found that compared with the usual care group, there were no significant differences in LOS (6.1 days per patient) compared with the usual care group (6.3 days per patient; P = .26) or hospital cost (US\$5640 and US\$5754; P = .68).[12]

Although the Counsel and colleagues RCT did not produce much influence on ADLs and LOS, process-of-care measures such as an increase in care plan use, physical therapy consultations, and improved satisfaction from patients, staff, and physicians were an unexpected benefit.[12] A third RCT by Landerfeld and colleagues in 1998 also concluded that no significant difference in patient functioning was observed using the ACE model.[13] Still, in this trial, LOS and cost were significantly lower, as well as the rate of hospital readmissions. There was little published literature during the 1990s related to hospital costs. The Landerfeld and colleagues RCT only received publication as an abstract, providing observational data.[13] Barnes and colleagues, also using an RCT in a community-setting hospital some 12 years later, sought to examine the effects of the ACE model on 1,632 patients aged 70 years and older during the more fiscal-minded era of the twenty-first century.[14] The researchers found that LOS was significantly reduced in the experimental group using the ACE model (6.7 days per patient) compared with the control group (7.3 days per patient). They hypothesized that the ACE model and the then-evolving hospitalist culture of caring for the geriatric population could reduce LOS and cost. In the Barnes and colleagues study, LOS and cost were highly correlated with each other (r = 0:91).

Starting in the late 90s, geriatric care in the acute care setting of hospitals in the US became increasingly relegated to general, internal medicine physicians, also known as hospitalists. Kuo and colleagues found that between 1995 and 2006, growth in hospitalists within the US increased from 5.9% to 19.0%, and claims for in-patient evaluation and management by hospitalists increased from 9.1% to 30.1%.[15] During the same period, Medicare patients treated by hospitalists increased from 46.4% to 61.0%.[15] Treatment delivered during hospitalization by hospitalists has been associated with shorter LOS and lower hospital costs.[16] This was a perfect storm of events: the emergence of the ACE model coincided with a growing hospitalist movement.

As with the first 3 studies implementing the ACE model of care, not only did the Barnes and colleagues study produce decreases in LOS and costs but also no significant differences were found between the ACE model group and the control group when it came to functioning at discharge; neither were there significant differences in discharges home versus discharge to an institution.[15] By the time the Barnes RCT concluded, the Center for Medicare and Medicaid Innovation began basing reimbursements on patients' total episodes of care instead of services provided. This meant the postdischarge costs associated with home health and rehabilitative services would have negatively influenced their cost findings.[16] It must also be mentioned that the Barnes RCT did not replicate the functional improvement of the previous studies. This finding was attributed to the study hospital's adoption of many of the original ACE protocols, such as skin care assessments and reduced use of restraints in the "usual care" group. It was also presumed that staff changes, including in leadership, led to a loss of fidelity within the control group over time.[15]

Evidence supporting the ACE unit model's benefit in reducing LOS, costs, and 30-day readmissions is strong within the literature. In an era when cost reduction and quality of care are important objectives of the Medicare program, the ACE unit model meets these goals.[17] The first ACE unit models focused primarily on reducing incidences of functional disability during acute hospitalizations for older adults. This included incorporating environmental room modifications necessary for older patients. During the early trials, the enhancement of the physical environment of the geriatric patient focused on independence and safety. Room modification became a major limitation to the startup of an ACE unit. Retraining professionals in the ACE unit model approach and remodeling rooms on a nursing unit proved challenging when considering corporate buy-in, even when cost savings were shown to exist through patient outcomes. Over time, a new movement evolved in the structural designs of newer community hospitals, heralding a newer structural design to patient rooms that are today similar to the prepared environment envisioned by the Cleveland group. Ushered in by patient-centered care models and Hospital Consumer Assessment of Healthcare Providers and Systems scores, many of today's nursing units are designed with ergonomics focused on the geriatric patient, such as designs to aid patients with impaired depth perception.[2]

With today's hospitalized geriatric patients living longer and increasingly more fragile, and with the positive outcomes offered by several ACE model unit trials, this model of care for older hospitalized patients would be expected to be adopted by every acute care hospital across the US but this has not been the case. Rogers and colleagues,[18] in 2020, surveyed 3692 hospitals across the US to assess the use of the ACE unit model and found that of 3692 hospitals surveyed, only 2055 responded (56%). More responses were from Urban hospitals (75%) than rural hospitals (25%). Of the 2055 respondents, 68 (3.3%) of hospitals identified as having or previously having an ACE unit, only 50 (2.4%) completed the entire survey. Seven of the 50 who completed the entire survey had closed their ACE units (14%), with 43 (86%) still operational.[18]

Limitations acknowledged by the Roger and colleagues study included having a small sample of hospitals complete the survey, not knowing who was filling out the survey (if they were a leader or implementer of the ACE unit), conducting the surveys during the 2020 winter surge of the coronavirus disease 2019 pandemic, and the lack of testing for reliability and validity of the survey instrument.[18]

The ACE Unit approach was not the first attempt to improve the quality of care for geriatric patients or the overall cost-effectiveness of care. During the 1970s, with mounting evidence that hospitals were unprepared for an increase of older, sicker adults enrolling in Medicare, several geriatric models of care began to emerge, focused on providing geriatric principles to reduce nosocomial complications to older adults. These models from the past included the geriatric resource nurse (GRN) model, the Geriatric Consultation service, the Hospital Elder Life Program, and the Advanced Practice Nurse Transitional Care model.[18] More recently was the Acute Care for Elders (ACE) unit and the NICHE program. Each model set out to target the same principles: educating health-care providers on geriatric principles, reducing nosocomial complications, and including the family in the plan of care.[19] To achieve these principles, one model sought not only to target these principles with interventions similar to the others (evidence-based, age-sensitive care) but also to emphasize educating those on the front line to care for the aging adults, the nurses.

The Nurses Improving Care for Health System Elders Program

The NICHE program was created in 1992 with the objective of improving system-level structures to support the clinical care of older adult patients and achieve better patient outcomes through goal-oriented strategies.[20] Created as a nurse-led institutional program providing consultation for hospitals caring for older adults, leadership training was the first step in organizational membership. Educating front-line clinical staff in mentoring and providing resources to assist nurses to critically think about strategies to care for older adult patients is the premise of the NICHE program. Similar to the ACE Unit model, NICHE uses an interprofessional approach to caring for older adult patients. After leadership training is complete, a multidimensional GRN model is created under the direction of NICHE consultants. The GRN model uses continuing education to create unit-based leaders in geriatric care through education, clinical rounds, and consultation with NICHE program consultants.[21]

The GRN is the gerontological nurse expert that drives the clinical team and coordinates a systematic approach to care for the older adult patient. Historically, a lack of formal training among nurses has hindered the development of care strategies for older adult patients.[21] Nurses are mentored to complete GRN educational modules and obtain national certification as gerontological nurses. Health systems participating in NICHE membership are offered an array of resources that strengthen the gerontological expertise of individual nurses and the health system's capacity to develop, use, and evaluate best practices in geriatric care.[22] Health systems interested in NICHE membership are encouraged to send at least 3 staff members to the 2-day NICHE leadership conference. There, the nurses are introduced to the NICHE tool kit, which includes clinical materials and resources to shape and support a system-wide transformation toward improved care of older adult patients.[22]

The NICHE Tool kit includes the health system's Geriatric Institutional Assessment Profile (GIAP). The GIAP is a 68-item questionnaire that assesses the health system staff's attitudes and knowledge about caring for older adult patients. This information is used by NICHE consultants to compare data against similar-sized health systems in similar demographics. NICHE consultants offer 4 nursing models for implementing best practices in geriatric care: the GRN model,[23] the ACE unit model,[24] the Comprehensive Discharge Planning/Quality Cost Model of Transitional Care,[25] and the Geriatric Syndrome Management Model.[26] A total of 14 best practice protocols are used within the NICHE program,[27] and a day-to-day manager is designated by the health-care facility to liaison with NICHE consultants—the NICHE coordinator.

Mezey and colleagues,[28,] in examining the characteristics of NICHE coordinators, found that of the 85 NICHE coordinators that returned surveys, 98% (n = 83) were women with a mean age of 47 years. Most (81%, n = 69) had master's degrees, 8% (n = 7) had doctoral degrees, and 40% (n = 34) were advanced practice, geriatric nurse practitioners or geriatric clinical nurse specialists. Nearly two-thirds (63%, n = 54) had direct care responsibilities, with most having some administrative responsibilities. Eighteen (23%) spent most of their time in administrative duties.[28]

The NICHE listserv connects NICHE coordinators to one another and the NICHE resource center at New York University's (NYU) Division of Nursing. Using the listserv, coordinators can ask and answer questions about practice protocols, research findings, procedures, and benchmarking. Membership in NICHE allows coordinators access to organizational and educational material to supplement the various models and protocols offered through the NICHE program. This includes the *Try This: Best Practices in Care for Older Adults* series offered by the Hartford Institute for Geriatric Nursing at NYU. The *Try This* series of screening tools aims to equip the clinician with a repertoire of best practices topics and instruments to care for older adults.[29]

The NICHE program has been successfully implemented within the ICU, improving health outcomes in older adults and their families.[30,31] Despite the evidence, hospitals, health-care systems, and provider organizations have not shown widespread adoption of the NICHE program.[32] In examining what factors did attribute to NICHE program adoption, Stimpfel and Gilmartin[33] used an observational, retrospective design to uncover statistically significant variables associated with hospital adoption of the NICHE program. The researchers used 3 conceptual models borrowed from organization and management theories to guide their selection of hospital and community characteristics favoring NICHE program adoption: the Market model, the Organizational-Managerial model, and the Sociotechnical model. Sampling 3506 NICHE hospitals between 2012 and 2013 and only including adult acute care hospitals, the researchers found that, first, NICHE hospitals were larger than non-NICHE hospitals (318 vs 146 beds: average). More NICHE hospitals were in urban areas (91% vs 53%). More NICHE hospitals were not-for-profit (80% vs 60%) than non-NICHE hospitals, NICHE hospitals had more specialized units for older adults than non-NICHE hospitals (64% vs 39%), and hospitals with more pain management programs were more likely to adopt the NICHE program (85% vs 53%).[33]

Barriers to Dissemination

During the last 3 decades, the ACE unit model and the NICHE program membership models have been studied and shown to improve care quality and increase overall cost-effectiveness. With the complexity of both models, they may not be widely disseminated or utilized because they face common market barriers: financial cost and benefits, organizational culture, and other external pressures from the market.[19] The ACE model and the NICHE program do not reduce costs so much as they provide clinical benefits with no increased cost.[24,28]

We have learned that the functional improvement of older adult patients seen in the earlier ACE trials was not repeated in later studies. The emphasis on lowering costs during acute stays and decreasing readmissions has become the focal point of current studies of these models. The original goal of reducing functional disability using the

ACE unit model seems to have been replaced by preserving the quality of care for older adult patients.

SUMMARY

The use of the ACE unit model and the NICHE program is sparse across US hospitals and health systems. During the past 30 years, 2 things have changed; the older adult patient is getting chronologically older and living longer, and the cost of caring for this population is getting higher. We may not see more of these evidence-based geriatric models because it is difficult to demonstrate cost savings in terms of cost avoidance. With a true ACE unit, there is an expected initial outlay of funds to redesign a unit with ACE specifications. Making the financial pitch to the medical facility's board of directors on converting to an ACE model or NICHE program for the ICU may prove difficult in an industry concerned with financial risk.

With both models, there is a need for a geriatric specialist. Within the NICHE program model, it would require time to grow the GRNs needed to implement the program. Implementing the ACE model would require hiring geriatric specialists, such as Geriatric Nurse Practitioners, from a small pool of providers in today's market. Quality and cost benchmarks are the driving force behind accountable care organization initiatives. Maybe, these models continue to exist as hybrids or as combinations of several models across US healthcare systems. Organizations may use these models' outcome data today to inform their practice protocols. The question remains, are we still using these geriatric models of care, and are they reducing costs in critical care?

CLINICS CARE POINTS

- Geriatric syndromes, such as hospital-acquired disability in older adults, are multifactorial.
- ACE units use an interdisciplinary rather than a multidisciplinary model to deliver care.
- The NICHE Model seeks to improve healthcare systems' delivery of quality care to older adults through nurse leadership and education.
- Older adults admitted to the hospital usually come with chronic illnesses into an unfamiliar and often restrictive environment.

DISCLOSURE

The author has no commercial or financial conflicts of interest or any sources of funding in writing this article

REFERENCES

1. Schimmel EM. The hazards of hospitalization. 1964. Qual Saf Health Care 2003; 12(1):58–64.
2. Palmer RM. The acute care for elders unit model of care. Geriatrics 2018;3(3):59.
3. Institute of Medicine Committee on Quality of Health Care in America. In: Kohn LT, Corrigan JM, Donaldson MS, editors. To Err is human: building a safer health system. Washington, DC: National Academies Press (US); 2000.
4. Brown CJ. After three decades of study, hospital-associated disability remains a common problem. J Am Geriatr Soc 2020;68(3):465–6.

5. Covinsky KE, Pierluissi E, Johnston CB. Hospitalization-associated disability: "She was probably able to ambulate, but I'm not sure". JAMA 2011;306(16): 1782–93.

6. Gill TM, Allore HG, Gahbauer EA, et al. Change in disability after hospitalization or restricted activity in older persons. JAMA 2010;304(17):1919–28 [published correction appears in JAMA. 2011;305(13):1301].

7. Chandra A, Dalton MA, Holmes J. Large increases in spending on post-acute care in Medicare point to the potential for cost savings in these settings. Health Aff 2013;32(5):864–72.

8. American Hospital Association, Fact Sheet: Post-Acute Care. Available at: https://www.aha.org/system/files/media/file/2019/07/fact-sheet-post-acute-care-0719.pdf. Accessed February 21, 2023.

9. Covinsky KE, Palmer RM, Fortinsky RH, et al. Loss of independence in activities of daily living in older adults hospitalized with medical illnesses: increased vulnerability with age. J Am Geriatr Soc 2003;51(4):451–8.

10. Cleveland J. Acute Care for Elders units: a model from the past or for the future? J Am Geriatr Soc 2022;70(10):2758–60.

11. Landefeld CS, Palmer RM, Kresevic DM, et al. A randomized trial of care in a hospital medical unit especially designed to improve the functional outcomes of acutely ill older patients. N Engl J Med 1995;332(20):1338–44.

12. Counsell SR, Holder CM, Liebenauer LL, et al. Effects of a multicomponent intervention on functional outcomes and process of care in hospitalized older patients: a randomized controlled trial of Acute Care for Elders (ACE) in a community hospital. J Am Geriatr Soc 2000;48(12):1572–81.

13. Landefeld CS, Palmer RM, Fortinsky RH, et al. A randomized trial of Acute Care for Elders (ACE) in the current era: lower hospital costs without adverse effects on functional outcomes at discharge. J Gen Intern Med 1998;13(suppl):45.

14. Barnes DE, Palmer RM, Kresevic DM, et al. Acute care for elders units produced shorter hospital stays at lower cost while maintaining patients' functional status. Health Aff 2012;31(6):1227–36.

15. Kuo YF, Sharma G, Freeman JL, et al. Growth in the care of older patients by hospitalists in the United States. N Engl J Med 2009;360(11):1102–12.

16. Center for Medicare and Medicaid Innovation. Bundled payments for care improvement Internet. Updated November 8, 2022.Accessed March 20, 2023. Available at: https://innovation.cms.gov/innovation-models/bundled-payments.

17. Flood KL, Maclennan PA, McGrew D, et al. Effects of an acute care for elders unit on costs and 30-day readmissions. JAMA Intern Med 2013;173(11):981–7.

18. Rogers SE, Flood KL, Kuang QY, et al. The current landscape of Acute Care for Elders units in the United States. J Am Geriatr Soc 2022;70(10):3012–20.

19. Capezuti E, Brush BL. Implementing geriatric care models: what are we waiting for? Geriatr Nurs 2009;30(3):204–6.

20. Squires A, Murali KP, Greenberg SA, et al. A scoping review of the evidence about the nurses improving care for healthsystem elders (NICHE) program. Gerontol 2021;61(3):e75–84.

21. Berman A, Mezey M, Kobayashi M, et al. Gerontological nursing content in baccalaureate nursing programs: comparison of findings from 1997 and 2003. J Prof Nurs 2005;21(5):268–75.

22. Boltz M, Harrington C, Kluger M. Nurses improving care for health system elders (NICHE). Am J Nurs 2005;105(5):101–2.

23. Rosenfeld P, Kwok G, Glassman K. Assessing the perceptions and attitudes among geriatric resource nurses: evaluating the NICHE program at a large academic medical center. Gerontol Geriatr Educ 2018;39(3):268–82.
24. Flood KL, Booth K, Vickers J, et al. Acute care for elders (ACE) team model of care: a clinical overview. Geriatrics 2018;3(3):50.
25. Naylor MD, Brooten D, Campbell R, et al. Comprehensive discharge planning and home follow-up of hospitalized elders: a randomized clinical trial. JAMA 1999;281(7):613–20.
26. Foreman MD, Wykle M. Nursing standard-of-practice protocol: sleep disturbances in elderly patients. The NICHE Faculty. Geriatr Nurs 1995;16(5):238–43.
27. Mezey M, Fulmer T, Abraham I, editors. Geriatric nursing protocols for best practice. 2nd ed. New York: Springer; 2003.
28. Mezey M, Kobayashi M, Grossman S, et al. Nurses improving care to health system elders (NICHE): implementation of best practice models. J Nurs Adm 2004; 34(10):451–7.
29. Hartford Institute for Geriatric Nursing (HIGN). Try This Series. Available at: https://hign.org/consultgeri-resources/try-this-series. Accessed March 29, 2023.
30. Boltz M, Capezuti E, Shuluk J, et al. Implementation of geriatric acute care best practices: initial results of the NICHE SITE self-evaluation. Nurs Health Sci 2013; 15(4):518–24.
31. Giambattista L, Howard R, Ruhe Porto R, et al. NICHE recommended care of the critically ill older adult. Crit Care Nurs Q 2015;38(3):223–30.
32. Malone ML, Capezuti E, Palmer RM, editors. Geriatrics models of care: bringing "best practice." to an aging America. New York: Springer; 2007.
33. Stimpfel AW, Gilmartin MJ. Factors predicting adoption of the nurses improving care of healthsystem elders program. Nurs Res 2019;68(1):13–21.

Moving?

Make sure your subscription moves with you!

To notify us of your new address, find your **Clinics Account Number** (located on your mailing label above your name), and contact customer service at:

Email: journalscustomerservice-usa@elsevier.com

800-654-2452 (subscribers in the U.S. & Canada)
314-447-8871 (subscribers outside of the U.S. & Canada)

Fax number: 314-447-8029

Elsevier Health Sciences Division
Subscription Customer Service
3251 Riverport Lane
Maryland Heights, MO 63043

*To ensure uninterrupted delivery of your subscription, please notify us at least 4 weeks in advance of move.

ELSEVIER

UNITED STATES POSTAL SERVICE ® Statement of Ownership, Management, and Circulation
(All Periodicals Publications Except Requester Publications)

1. Publication Title	2. Publication Number	3. Filing Date
CRITICAL CARE NURSING CLINICS OF NORTH AMERICA	006 – 273	9/18/23

4. Issue Frequency	5. Number of Issues Published Annually	6. Annual Subscription Price
MAR, JUN SEP, DEC	4	$160.00

7. Complete Mailing Address of Known Office of Publication (Not printer) (Street, city, county, state, and ZIP+4®)

ELSEVIER INC.
230 Park Avenue, Suite 800
New York, NY 10169

Contact Person
Malathi Samayan

Telephone (Include area code)
91-44-4299-4507

8. Complete Mailing Address of Headquarters or General Business Office of Publisher (Not printer)

ELSEVIER INC.
230 Park Avenue, Suite 800
New York, NY 10169

9. Full Names and Complete Mailing Addresses of Publisher, Editor, and Managing Editor (Do not leave blank)

Publisher (Name and complete mailing address)

DOLORES MELONI, ELSEVIER INC.
1600 JOHN F KENNEDY BLVD. SUITE 1600
PHILADELPHIA, PA 19103-2899

Editor (Name and complete mailing address)

KERRY HOLLAND, ELSEVIER INC.
1600 JOHN F KENNEDY BLVD. SUITE 1600
PHILADELPHIA, PA 19103-2899

Managing Editor (Name and complete mailing address)

PATRICK MANLEY, ELSEVIER INC.
1600 JOHN F KENNEDY BLVD. SUITE 1600
PHILADELPHIA, PA 19103-2899

10. Owner (Do not leave blank. If the publication is owned by a corporation, give the name and address of the corporation immediately followed by the names and addresses of all stockholders owning or holding 1 percent or more of the total amount of stock. If not owned by a corporation, give the names and addresses of the individual owners. If owned by a partnership or other unincorporated firm, give its name and address as well as those of each individual owner. If the publication is published by a nonprofit organization, give its name and address.)

Full Name	Complete Mailing Address
WHOLLY OWNED SUBSIDIARY OF REED/ELSEVIER, US HOLDINGS	1600 JOHN F KENNEDY BLVD. SUITE 1600 PHILADELPHIA, PA 19103-2899

11. Known Bondholders, Mortgagees, and Other Security Holders Owning or Holding 1 Percent or More of Total Amount of Bonds, Mortgages, or Other Securities. If none, check box ▶ ☐ None

Full Name	Complete Mailing Address
N/A	

12. Tax Status (For completion by nonprofit organizations authorized to mail at nonprofit rates) (Check one)
The purpose, function, and nonprofit status of this organization and the exempt status for federal income tax purposes:
☒ Has Not Changed During Preceding 12 Months
☐ Has Changed During Preceding 12 Months (Publisher must submit explanation of change with this statement)

PS Form **3526**, July 2014 [Page 1 of 4 (see instructions page 4)] PSN: 7530-01-000-9931   PRIVACY NOTICE: See our privacy policy on www.usps.com.

---

13. Publication Title	14. Issue Date for Circulation Data Below
CRITICAL CARE NURSING CLINICS OF NORTH AMERICA	JUNE 2023

15. Extent and Nature of Circulation		Average No. Copies Each Issue During Preceding 12 Months	No. Copies of Single Issue Published Nearest to Filing Date
a. Total Number of Copies (Net press run)		85	89
b. Paid Circulation (By Mail and Outside the Mail)	(1) Mailed Outside-County Paid Subscriptions Stated on PS Form 3541 (Include paid distribution above nominal rate, advertiser's proof copies, and exchange copies)	50	49
	(2) Mailed In-County Paid Subscriptions Stated on PS Form 3541 (Include paid distribution above nominal rate, advertiser's proof copies, and exchange copies)	0	0
	(3) Paid Distribution Outside the Mails Including Sales Through Dealers and Carriers, Street Vendors, Counter Sales, and Other Paid Distribution Outside USPS®	20	20
	(4) Paid Distribution by Other Classes of Mail Through the USPS (e.g., First-Class Mail®)	7	12
c. Total Paid Distribution (Sum of 15b (1), (2), (3), and (4))	▶	77	81
d. Free or Nominal Rate Distribution (By Mail and Outside the Mail)	(1) Free or Nominal Rate Outside-County Copies included on PS Form 3541	7	7
	(2) Free or Nominal Rate In-County Copies Included on PS Form 3541	0	0
	(3) Free or Nominal Rate Copies Mailed at Other Classes Through the USPS (e.g., First-Class Mail)	0	0
	(4) Free or Nominal Rate Distribution Outside the Mail (Carriers or other means)	1	1
e. Total Free or Nominal Rate Distribution (Sum of 15d (1), (2), (3) and (4))	▶	8	8
f. Total Distribution (Sum of 15c and 15e)	▶	85	89
g. Copies not Distributed (See Instructions to Publishers #4 (page #3))	▶	0	0
h. Total (Sum of 15f and g)		85	89
i. Percent Paid (15c divided by 15f times 100)		90.56%	91.01%

* If you are claiming electronic copies, go to line 16 on page 3. If you are not claiming electronic copies, skip to line 17 on page 3.

16. Electronic Copy Circulation		Average No. Copies Each Issue During Preceding 12 Months	No. Copies of Single Issue Published Nearest to Filing Date
a. Paid Electronic Copies	▶		
b. Total Paid Print Copies (Line 15c) + Paid Electronic Copies (Line 16a)	▶		
c. Total Print Distribution (Line 15f) + Paid Electronic Copies (Line 16a)	▶		
d. Percent Paid (Both Print & Electronic Copies) (16b divided by 16c × 100)	▶		

☒ I certify that 50% of all my distributed copies (electronic and print) are paid above a nominal price.

17. Publication of Statement of Ownership
☒ If the publication is a general publication, publication of this statement is required. Will be printed ☐ Publication not required.
in the DECEMBER 2023 issue of this publication.

18. Signature and Title of Editor, Publisher, Business Manager, or Owner

Malathi Samayan - Distribution Controller

Malathi Samayan

Date 9/18/23

I certify that all information furnished on this form is true and complete. I understand that anyone who furnishes false or misleading information on this form or who omits material or information requested on the form may be subject to criminal sanctions (including fines and imprisonment) and/or civil sanctions (including civil penalties).

PS Form **3526**, July 2014 (Page 3 of 4)   PRIVACY NOTICE: See our privacy policy on www.usps.com

9780443131011